Management of Back Pain

Management of Back Pain

Richard W. Porter MD FRCS FRCSE
Consultant Orthopaedic Surgeon
Doncaster Royal Infirmary
Doncaster UK

Contributor

Paul Butt MD FRCR FRCP(C)
Consultant Radiologist
St James University Hospital
Leeds UK

CHURCHILL LIVINGSTONE
EDINBURGH LONDON MELBOURNE AND NEW YORK 1986

CHURCHILL LIVINGSTONE
Medical Division of Longman Group Limited

Distributed in the United States of America by Churchill
Livingstone Inc., 1560 Broadway, New York, N.Y. 10036, and
by associated companies, branches and representatives
throughout the world.

First published 1986

ISBN 0 443 02954 7

British Library Cataloguing in Publication Data
Porter, R.W.
  Management of back pain.
  1. Backache
  I. Title
  616.7'3   RD768

Library of Congress Cataloging in Publication Data
Porter, R. W. (Richard William)
  Management of back pain
  Includes index.
  1. Backache. 1. Title. [DNLM: 1. Backache.
WE 755 P847m]
RD768.P677 1985   617'.56   85–19513

Printed in Great Britain
at the University Printing House, Oxford

Preface

It is not an easy task to write a book about back pain, when one is more aware of our ignorance than our knowledge. Back pain is but a symptom. The possible causes are legion, some of which we find, and some elude us. But the quest lends a fascination that I hope is reflected in these chapters.

The book falls naturally into three sections. We start with the basic sciences, then recognisable back pain syndromes with their management, and finally ways in which back pain may be prevented. 'Management' is a more appropriate word than 'treatment', the latter suggesting therapy that will lead to a cure. With backs this is rarely possible, and even following surgery a cure is relative. Management means sharing with the patients an understanding of the source of pain, and how the natural history of the condition can be used to their advantage, rather than be aggravated by miscalculated daily activity and misplaced therapy. Management is the art of the possible; cures are a little more difficult.

I remember a preacher friend telling me that he always tried to be informative, interesting and inspiring. I hope that you will find these qualities here. Information about backs has exploded in recent years and I pass on in a constructed form what I have learnt from others. Like Paul the apostle, I am a debtor. Backs are interesting when we apply all the available knowledge to unravel the diagnostic riddle of 'what is wrong?', and more so as we curiously ask: 'what is the mechanism of that patient's behaviour?'.

But we need more. We need a breath of inspiration if our understanding of back pain is to move forward. Some of our steps when tested will be proved wrong, but try we must. The quest has barely started. The history of back pain matches the history of man, and we have only just begun to ask 'Why?'. To think we have made more than the first faltering steps would be presumptuous. Inspiration means freedom to be original, and if there are any new concepts in this book, they are to be tested by experience.

The untimely death of Bill Parke has robbed us of his help in Chapter 8, 'Radiological investigation', but we quote his writings and include his concepts.

No treatise on the subject can be universally acceptable, when the spectrum of opinion is so wide. Neither can it be comprehensive. I have not described in detail surgical technique, nor have I dealt in depth with back pain of inflammatory origin. One can only describe the view from where you are, and mine is an orthopaedic vantage, assisted by my good friend and radiologist, Paul Butt. I hope it will complement the work of other disciplines, stimulate thought, help us move forwards, and ultimately be of value to the patient with the painful back.

Doncaster, 1986   R.W.P.

Acknowledgements

I would like to thank Armour Pharmaceutical Ltd for their financial assistance in producing the figures; the opinions I have expressed do not necessarily reflect their views. Thanks too for Mr Garry Swann's help in the photography, and to Mrs Jean Reynolds for her secretarial assistance. And of course thanks for the tolerance of Christine, Daniel, William, Matthew and James.

Contents

1

Back pain — a problem — personal, national and clinical

Back pain is a national, personal and clinical problem; national because it is experienced by most of the population at some time and is a drain on the nation's resources; personal because it can remain a major unresolved dilemma and clinical because not only is diagnosis difficult, but methods of treatment are conflicting and often unrewarding.

A PERSONAL PROBLEM

For the patient, back pain is more than an academic manipulation of statistics; it is a personal problem of epidemic proportions. It causes half the population to seek help from their general practitioner at some time (Jayson, 1981). The incidence of attendance varies from 20 to 37 per thousand per year (Fry, 1974, Lewith and Turner, 1982, Drinkall et al, 1984), and about one visit in four is a first attendance for back pain.

Attendance depends not only on the incidence of back pain, but the ethos of the community (Bremner et al, 1968) and the management of the practice. We examined over eight hundred records of 40 year old men and their wives from four South Yorkshire practices, and over a twenty year period, 50–81 per cent of the men and 26–63 per cent of the women attended at some time with back pain (Table 1.1).

By the time the doctor is approached it is more than the touch of back pain that we can all expect from time to time. It has become unmanageable, interfering with mobility, work, sleep and recreation. The high male incidence especially in the fifth decade (Wood and McLeish, 1974) may not reflect the true perspective. Women, the young and the elderly may be less inclined to seek help. Fin Biering-Sorensen (1982) recorded an increasing incidence amongst women in advancing years.

Table 1.1 Percentage of 40 year old men and their wives who attended their general practitioner at some time in the previous twenty years with low back pain. (n = 855)

	% of men who attended with back pain	% of their wives who attended with low low back pain	% of men who were heavy manual workers
Practice A	81	54	49
Practice B	65	26	65
Practice C	62	63	18
Practice D	50	39	22

General practice statistics underestimate the problem. Half the patients treated by registered osteopaths have back pain, and one in three of these have not seen their own doctor (Burton, 1978, 1981). For all of these back pain is a problem. A problem because of the severity of the pain, its persistence, its disabling effects, the fear of its origin, and apprehension about the future. Too often it is compounded by different practitioners offering various diagnoses or admitting ignorance, by recommending no treatment or contradictory methods. The patient is understandably confused, and for those whose pain does not settle naturally with time, anxiety or depression adds to their dilemma.

Mr G.S. was a dynamic sales representative who, at 35, was in charge of fifteen salesmen serving two counties. Out of the blue he found himself in bed with pain in the back and left leg and restricted straight leg raising. He failed to improve over three weeks. A lower lumbar disc was speedily excised but recovery was slow, and after three months, in spite of aching in the back and left leg, he forced himself back to work. For five years his employers were satisfied with him, but his wife and two boys suffered. No sex, no sports, no fun; Dad always seemed to be in some sort of pain. He couldn't even walk at a normal pace, and both legs seemed to tighten up after five minutes. He would rest, and walk further, but after a heavy day, his legs were so restless in bed he had to sleep in a room of his own. Some experts diagnosed spinal stenosis, and he agreed to have a spinal decompression, but now at 42 years of age, after a second operation, he still has very limited walking distance and episodes of back pain that put him to bed from time to time. He stands to lose his job.

Mrs G.N. is ten years older than her husband, and at 39 years of age she and her family think she should be able to run her home, engage in an active social life and have energetic holidays. For three years, however, she has had a painful back whenever she does heavy work. She has no sex life, and she fears for her marriage. Two months ago she spent a week lying on the floor, and all she can remember the orthopaedic surgeon saying to her as he could hardly raise either of her heels from the floor, was 'never mind dear, we all get back pain and you will have to live with it'.

Mr J McH is twenty six, plays professional soccer and is the club's best striker. He thought he had a hamstring strain, missed a few games, but when his ankle reflex was affected, he was soon in the hands of a surgeon and a prolapsed disc was removed. Now his pain has settled, but he has a weak soleus and cannot stand on his toes. The club cannot afford to renew his contract, and with no other work experience he has moved from the glare of the floodlights to the dole queue.

Mrs J.D. is sixty two, remembers having a couple of bad years with pain in the back and leg in her twenties, and has treated her back with respect ever since. For two years now she has had periods of severe pain in the right leg from the buttock, thigh, calf to the ankle. It is getting worse and now keeps her awake at night. Sometimes she takes twenty analgesics a day. She has had three epidural injections, with only temporary relief. She looks strained and nervous, prefers to stand rather than sit when she visits the clinic, and asks if an operation will help her.

Mr H.R. was a coal-face worker earning good money until his back began to ache after a heavy shift. Within six months it became a constant ache, relieved only by lying down. An X-ray showed a spondylolisthesis and he was advised to take a light job in the pit bottom. Even this proved too much until now he is not working at all. Not yet 40 years old, he sits at home whilst his wife goes out to work. He is trying to prove that a fall of coal strained his back and caused his problem, but cannot understand why the doctors say it would have been painful anyway. If he exagerrates a bit, it is only to convince the doctors there is really something wrong with him. They all seem to think he is malingering and no-one understands him. Even his wife says it must be 'in his mind'.

These histories are real, and in spite of expert medical help, the problems remain.

A NATIONAL PROBLEM

Viewed from a national perspective the problem is enormous. As many as 35 per cent of patients who visit their general practitioner with back pain may be in sufficient trouble to be referred at some time to hospital (Barker, 1977), (Table 1.2). This may be as much as nine per cent referral in any one year (Fig. 1.1). Orthopaedic surgeons and rheumatologists in the U.K. see 0.4 million patients per year with back pain (Jayson, 1981). Many of these have been waiting in excess of three months for an appointment, with months off work and little prospect of an early return. Their investigations absorb a large proportion of the radiological budget, and their management is a large

Table 1.2 Use of hospital resources for 40 year old men (n = 393) who had experienced some low back pain in the previous twenty years, in four general practices.

	% of men with low back pain referred for spinal radiographs	% of men with low back pain referred for orthopaedic opinion
Practice A	44	24
Practice B	23	21
Practice C	33	13
Practice D	37	35

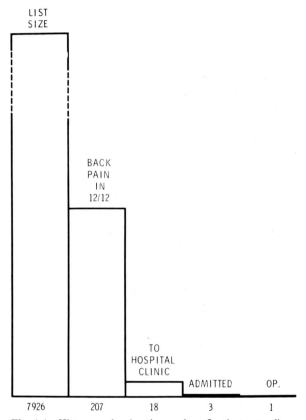

Fig. 1.1 Histogram showing the number of patients attending a general practice in a one year period complaining of low back pain and the number referred to hospital (Drinkall et al, 1984).

part of the workload of the physiotherapy and appliance departments.

Only a minority of patients will be offered surgery, with successes balanced by an equal number of failures. Up to 7500 disc operations are performed each year in Britain, 15 per 100 000 of the population. (There is more enthusiasm for disc surgery in the United States where 69.5 operations per 100 000 are performed each year, Nelson, 1983).

The cost of back pain to the National Health Service is currently £60 million per year (Cochrane, 1979). Social Security pays out at least £40 million per year in sickness and invalidity benefits and disablement pensions for back pain. The community loses about £220 million in lost output per year, and this is a gross underestimate. In the coal-mining industry, 11.9 per cent of certified absences is due to back pain (Afacan, 1982) and it can be argued that the loss to the industry of one face worker for a year is £100,000 mainly in lost production (MacDonald et al, 1984). The economic cost to the nation is staggering.

Heavy manual workers who are the main producers of the national wealth are those most likely to suffer back pain (Fig. 1.2). Seventy-five per cent of miners will have some back pain and most of those be off work with it at some time, whilst 50 per cent of office workers will experience back pain and half of them need to be off work, (Fig. 1.3). There is a high incidence of back pain amongst truck drivers (Kelsey, 1975), tractor drivers (Matthews, 1964a and b, Allawi, 1978), helicopter pilots, (Fitzgerald and Crotty, 1972), bricklayers, nurses in medical, geriatric and orthopaedic wards (Cust et al, 1972) and in those parts of an industry where heavy load handling is required (Troup, 1968, Chaffin and Park, 1973, Frymoyer et al, 1983). Measured in economic terms, back pain is probably the largest medical problem awaiting a solution.

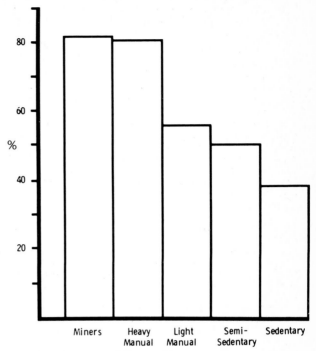

Fig. 1.2 Percentage of 40 year old men according to occupation who had previously visited their general practitioner with low back pain.

A CLINICAL PROBLEM

To the clinician, the problem is pertinent. Faced with a patient asking two questions, 'What is causing the

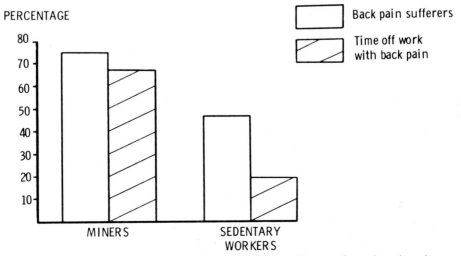

Fig. 1.3 Percentage of miners (n = 251) and sedentary workers (n = 198) over 50 years of age who at interview stated that they had experienced low back pain in the past and who had at some time been off work with low back pain.

back pain?' and 'Can you put it right?' it is often difficult to give a satisfactory answer to either.

In most medical conditions we seek a diagnosis. We listen and question the patient, examine and investigate, until we are satisfied we have identified the pathological condition which is responsible for the symptoms. We are satisfied even if we cannot be too sure how the symptoms are experienced by the patient. When investigating back pain, however, we are frequently uncertain which part of the spinal anatomy is sufficiently deranged to produce pain. All too often we cannot find the pain source. We have no diagnosis, and therefore a problem.

In the past clinicians have described back pain with ambiguous words like 'lumbago', 'fibrositis', 'slipped disc', as though providing a label was as good as a diagnosis. Other physicians have accepted our ignorance of the pain source, describing undiagnosed back pain as 'non specific back pain' (Jayson, 1984). Our very terminology confirms that all too frequently we have no diagnosis.

If the patient's first question is difficult, the second is no easier. How can you treat a problem when you don't know its cause? It is generally true that when a variety of remedies abound to treat a condition, there is no cure. For back pain this is certainly correct.

The methods of treatment are legion, from exercise to rest, manipulation to immobilisation; drugs by mouth, into muscles, into joints, discs, the spine; needles and knives; relaxation, stimulators, bending the mind and strengthening the faith. When it comes to a scientific appraisal of our efforts to treat back pain, it must be confessed that in the long term, no one method of treatment seems better than doing nothing at all (Nachemson, 1976).

Problems indeed for a clinician in a scientific age, when health expectations are high. No diagnosis and no treatment of proven worth. We are left with two choices, nihilism, despair and defeat, or a positive approach of facing up to the difficulties, clearing away the myths, and patiently seeking to answer questions from a base of known facts. The problems are great but so is the reward. Back pain can be one of the most interesting and stimulating fields of medicine. The reward of searching for a diagnosis, to find a pain source. The reward of a patient's gratitude that someone is sufficiently interested to try, and is prepared to give time, to listen and explain. The reward of combining with colleagues in so many disciplines, the bio-engineers, the bio-chemists, mathematicians, clinicians and therapists to answer some of the unsolved questions. The reward perhaps of reducing the back pain problem for a future generation. We can try.

REFERENCES

Afacan A S 1982 Sickness absence due to back lesions in coal miners. Journal of the Society of Occupational Medicine 32: 26–31

Allawi A 1978 Postmen with driving commitments have higher complaints about LBP than those without. Ph.D thesis, University of London

Barker M E 1977 Pain in the back and leg: a general practice survey

Bremner J M, Lawrence J S 1968. Degenerative joint disease in a Jamaican rural population. Annals of Rheumatic Diseases 27: 326–332

Burton A K 1978 The prior medical contact of osteopath's patients. British Osteopath Journal 11: 19–23

Burton A K 1981 Back pain in osteopathic practice. Rheumatology and Rehabilitation 20: 239–246

Chaffin D B, Park K S, 1973, A longitudinal study of low back pain as associated with occupational weight lifting factors. American Industrial Hyg. Ass. Journal, 34: 513–523.

Cochrane A L 1979 Working group on back pain. Report to secretary of state for social services, secretary of state for Scotland. London: Her Majesty's Stationary Office

Cust G, Pearson J C G, Mair A 1972 The prevalence of low back pain in nurses. International nursing review 19: 169–179

Drinkall J N, Porter R W, Hibbert C S, Evans C 1984 The value of ultrasonic measurement of the spinal canal diameter in general practice. British Medical Journal 288: 121–122

Fin Biering-Sorensen 1982 Low back trouble in a general population of 30- 40- 50- and 60-year old men and women. Danish Medical Bulletin 29: 289–299

Fitzgerald J G, Crotty J 1972 The incidence of backache among air crew and ground crew in the Royal Air Force. Flying Personnel Research Committee — Ministry of Defence (Air Force Department) FPRC/1313

Frymoyer J W, Pope M H, Clements J H, Wilder D G, MacPhearson B, Ashikaga T 1983. Risk factors in low back pain. Journal of Bone and Joint Surgery 65–A: 213–218

Fry J 1974 Common diseases: their nature, incidence and care. MTP Press Ltd. London

Jayson M I V 1981 Back pain: the facts. Oxford University Press. New York, Toronto

Jayson M I V 1984 Difficult diagnoses in back pain. British Medical Journal 288: 740–741

Kelsey J L 1975 An epidemiological study of acute herniated lumbar intervertebral discs. Rheumatology and Rehabilitation 14: 144–159.

Lewith G T, Turner G M T 1982 Retrospective analysis of the management of acute low back pain. Practitioner, 226: 1614–1618.

Macdonald E B, Porter R W, Hibbert C, Hart J 1984 The relationship between spinal canal diameter and back pain in coal miners: ultrasonic measurement as a screening test? Journal of Occupational Medicine 26: 23–28.

Matthews J 1964a Journal of Agricultural Engineering, Res. 9, 3

Matthews J 1964b Journal of Agricultural Engineering, Res. 9, 147

Nachemson A L 1976 The lumbar spine. An orthopaedic challenge. Spine 1: 59–84

Nelson M 1983 Orthopaedic surgery: proceedings of the international symposium on low back pain and industrial and social disablement, p.91, Back Pain Association

Troup J D G 1968 The function of the lumbar spine. Ph.D thesis, University of London

Wood P H N, McLeish C L 1974 Annals of Rheumatic Diseases, 33: 93–105

2

The causes of back pain: aetiology

Back pain is but a symptom and its source may arise in many different structures. Most who complain of back pain have a problem with either the spine, or associated structures, but back pain can of course be the presenting symptom of pathology in other systems, and perhaps we should discuss these first.

BACK PAIN FROM NON SPINAL CAUSES

Gynaecological causes account for the largest number of patients with back pain when spinal problems are excluded. Pain associated with menstruation is recognised with its periodicity and its constant nature over several hours and it is unrelated to posture and activity. Uterine prolapse, fibroids, or a retroverted uterus not infrequently produce low back pain, aggravated by standing and walking, and relieved by rest. When there is presumptive evidence of gynaecological pathology, one can usually exclude a spinal cause for the pain if there are no abnormal spinal signs — that is a good range of lumbar movement and no tenderness. Not infrequently the spine is restricted and tender, and it is difficult to exclude a coexistent spinal problem.

A few patients are referred after pelvic surgery still with their back pain, and it becomes obvious in retrospect that there is also a spinal problem. Some are referred with pain after treatment of a pelvic carcinoma in the hope that there is an innocuous mechanical problem. Too frequently the constant nature of the pain suggests a recurrence of the tumour.

Renal pain

It is not usually difficult to distinguish between renal pain and derangement of the upper lumbar spine. The kidney generally produces pain in the loin, an unusual site for spinal pain, and it tends to be constant, building up to a peak, gradually settling over several hours, and being unaffected by posture and activity. Ureteric pain can produce pain radiating into the iliac fossa and groin in the same distribution as a lower thoracic or upper lumbar root lesion, but it tends to be constant for several hours at a time. Frequency and dysuria support the diagnosis, and a full renal investigation is necessary.

Retroperitoneal pathology

Pancreatic lesions can produce back pain which may initially be thought to have a spinal cause. One becomes suspicious, if there is a short history of increasing discomfort, fairly constant in nature, and associated with loss of weight. Abdominal examination, which should never be omitted when examining a back, may still be unhelpful. A high Erythrocyte Sedimentation Rate will add to the suspicions but the diagnosis may require contrast radiography, ultrasound examination or even laparotomy. It may take a laparotomy to identify retroperitoneal fibrosis as a cause of back pain (Pryor et al, 1983).

Gall stones, cholecystitis, or retro-caecal appendicitis, can present with back pain, but the true pathology soon declares itself. An aneurism of the aorta may be missed if the abdomen is not examined. A slow dissection of an aneurism may produce acute back pain, put a patient to bed, and only examination of the abdomen and palpation and auscultation of the femoral arteries will avoid a mis-diagnosis.

OTHER CAUSES OF LEG PAIN

Peripheral nerve entrapment syndromes may be confused with root pain. Entrapment of the lateral popliteal nerve at the neck of the fibula produces severe pain in the front and outer side of the shin down to the outer ankle and dorsum of the foot. Weakness of dorsi flexion is not invariably present. The lateral popliteal nerve is very sensitive to palpation between the fingers and the neck of the fibula, and contrasts well with the opposite leg. The lesion is confirmed by nerve conduction studies, with increased latency and delayed conduction and decompression surgically gives relief.

Meralgia parasthetica, or entrapment of the lateral cutaneous nerve of the thigh, can cause unpleasant and at times severe pain in the outer thigh. There is little doubt about the diagnosis if the pain is localised only to the antero-lateral thigh, and especially if there is some blunting to sensation in this area. Posture often influences this pain, being worse when stretching out in bed, sitting in a chair, and being relieved by changing position. There is sometimes a history of some precipitating compression like wearing a tight girdle, or having had pelvic traction. Excision of a segment of the nerve medial to the anterior superior iliac spine relieves the pain but sometimes an explanation of the cause is sufficient to satisfy patients without recourse to surgery.

The posterior tibial nerve can be the source of symptoms in the foot from entrapment behind and distal to the medial malleolus. This Tarsal Tunnel Syndrome tends to produce discomfort, especially at rest and in bed at night. It is described as pins and needles or even pain, in the sole of the foot. It is frequently associated with pes planus, oedema or a previous fracture. Nerve conduction studies confirm delayed conduction, and decompression of the tarsal tunnel well distally into the sole of the foot gives relief.

Intermittent claudication from peripheral arterial disease may be confused with, or even associated with, neurogenic claudication. Ischaemic claudication usually has a consistent pain tolerance and is worse ascending a hill or stairs, whilst neurogenic claudication is worse when the spine is extended going down a slope. If the peripheral pulses are difficult to palpate, a doppler scan will confirm arterial patency. Femoral bruits on auscultation may be the only clinical sign of an arterial cause of leg pain.

Varicose veins can cause aching in the calves and feet when standing or walking, and cramp at night.

This is usually below the knee and diffuse, whilst lumbar root pain is in a root distribution and is rarely limited to the lower leg alone.

Acute infective polyneuritis (Guillain-Barre Syndrome) can present like an acute mechanical derangement of the spine. Normally the syndrome begins with headache, vomiting, pyrexia, and pain in the back and limbs, but the back pain can occasionally be the presenting feature with pain and weakness in the legs overshadowing other symptoms (Turek, 1976). A generalised problem is suspected when the leg pain is not in a single nerve root distribution, and especially when upper limb symptoms are present. The diagnosis may be delayed if pain or weakness in the upper limbs and if respiratory difficulty is dismissed as functional.

BACK PAIN FROM BONY PATHOLOGY

Secondary tumour deposits in the vertebrae tend to produce pain before they are radiologically detectable, the pain being constant, unrelated to posture, and steadily increasing in severity. Scintigraphy will confirm increased vascularity before radiological features are present on routine films but eventually the cancellous structures of the vertebrae, the bodies, pedicles and spinous processes show bony destruction (or occasionally osteosclerosis in some metastatic deposits from the prostate and breast). The common primaries are breast, prostate and kidney. The definitive pathological diagnosis must generally be based on histological (and bacteriological) examination of the affected tissue. A needle biopsy with a Warwick needle under local anaesthetic, image intensifyer control and the lateral approach (Warwick, 1970, McCulloch and Waddell, 1978) is relatively straightforward in the lumbar spine but it needs an experienced bone pathologist to provide dependable results.

Primary bone tumours are unusual in the spine though Paget's sarcoma, chordoma, osteoid osteoma, angiosarcoma, solitary myeloma, malignant lymphoma, reticulum cell sarcoma can occur. Osteoid osteoma and benign osteoblastoma of the vertebrae can present with back pain and a fixed scoliosis, a rare combination in children and adolescents with mechanical derangement only (Freiberger, 1960, Kirwan et al, 1984). This should cause close inspection of the pedicles at the apex of the curve.

The most useful and reliable investigations are a Technetium bone scan to determine the level of the lesion and a CAT scan to identify precise location of the nidus (Fig. 2.1).

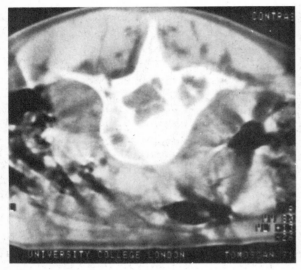

Fig. 2.1   CT scan demonstrating the nidus of an osteoid osteoma in the pedicle of L3 with surrounding bone sclerosis extending into the body, transverse process and lamina. (By kind permission of Mr. E. O'G. Kirwan.)

Small osteolytic deposits of multiple myelomatosis can be scattered through many bones causing back pain, and fractures associated with myelomatosis or with leukaemia will produce pain. All too frequently spinal bone tumours are not diagnosed until they produce neurological compression signs (Fig. 2.2). Unremitting pain and an absence of a previous history of back pain, especially in the elderly, should cause one to suspect malignancy. Simple angiomata of the vertebral bodies are usually symptomless, and discovered by chance on routine radiographs. On careful examination they can be recognised in 10 per cent of spines (Finneson, 1973), and perhaps should not be considered tumours at all. They do not require treatment. In fact, radiotherapy may result in osteoporosis and vertebral collapse (Roaf, 1980).

Tumours within the vertebral canal can cause pain with or without neurological signs. Extra medullary tumours such as neurofibromas, angiomas, lipomas, meningiomas, may cause compressive lesions of the cauda equina. Neurofibromata can enlarge the intervertebral foramen from bone erosion and cause root pain.

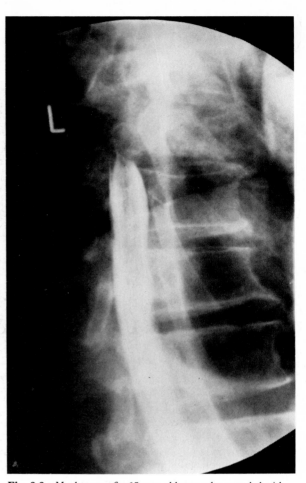

Fig. 2.2   Myelogram of a 65 year old man who attended with an unsteady gait showing occlusion of the metrizamide column at the upper border of D10. There is a compression fracture of D9 with sclerosis from a secondary deposit of a prostatic carcinoma.

Vertebral osteomyelitis is most commonly caused by haematogenous spread of *S. aureus,* although a wide range of other bacteria have been isolated including coliforms, pseudomonas, streptococci, brucella and mycobacterium tuberculosis, fungi and anaerobes. Infection can be introduced during spinal surgery, during epidural injections, myelography, or it can spread from adjacent lesions (Farrington et al, 1983, Digby and Kersley, 1979). It is not always easily differentiated from mechanical causes of back pain on clinical grounds alone. An acute pyogenic osteomyelitis of the vertebral body may be superimposed on a pre-existing back problem. Pain is aggravated by activity and relieved by rest. There is frequently a great deal of muscle spasm, more than is usually encountered with an acute disc lesion (Rae et al, 1984). Pyrexia, loss of weight and loss of appetite accompany spinal infection but all too frequently spinal infection is not suspected until a late stage (Flood et al, 1983). It may present as abdominal pain, or be associated with other debilitating illness like diabetes. The radiological features of vertebral osteomyelitis are characterisitic, with destruction of the end-plate, and disc space narrowing. The avascular discs are soon involved and rapidly destroyed by proteolytic enzymes of the pyogenic exudate with spread to the adjacent vertebrae. Tuberculosis on the other hand, tends to spread to the next vertebra around the disc under the anterior longitudinal ligament. Similarly in spinal neoplasms, the discs are generally preserved.

Whilst haematogenous osteomyelitis of the long bones is more common in children, vertebral osteomyelitis is decidedly rare under nine years of age (Allen et al, 1978). The highest incidence is in the third decade, probably because in adults and adolescents the lumbar intra-osseous arteries are end arteries, supplying a segment of bone. In children there is an extensive intra-osseous arterial anastomotic network (Ratcliffe, 1982).

Spinal tuberculosis is now fortunately a rare condition in Britain. Its previously common involvement of many vertebrae with collapse of the bodies and cold abscess formation is now unusual. The vertebral bodies were commonly affected, often a whole segment of the vertebral column, with progressive destruction of the cancellous bone, vertebral collapse and spread to adjacent vertebrae under the anterior longitudinal ligament. The discs were usually resistant, disappearing at a late stage. Cord involvement was a complication to be feared. It is, however, becoming an occasional disease of the elderly, particularly men (Horne, 1984). Now its presentation and features can be much the same as pyogenic osteomyelitis (Lichyenstein, 1975) and it is distinguished only by identification of the causative organism.

Spinal epidural abscess is encountered rarely, but should be considered when compressive symptoms are associated with severe pain. There is often a co-existing debilitating disease like diabetes or cirrhosis, and a source of infection from spinal surgery, needle investigation, or even retroperitoneal surgery (Russell et al, 1979).

INFLAMMATORY CAUSES OF BACK PAIN

Having described causes of back pain from non-spinal pathology and back pain associated with tumour and infection, there remain two broad categories of back pain affecting the spine, inflammatory and mechanical.

Back pain related to an inflammatory disorder is more common in young men, is worse after rest, improves with exercise, tends to be episodic, is referred from the low back to one or other buttock or posterior thigh, but not commonly to both at the same time, and there is often a history of other joint involvement (Calin, 1979). There may be a history of urethritis, uvulitis, psoriasis, ulcerative colitis or gout.

Ankylosing spondylitis in its severe form is easily recognised. The spine is stiff, too often in the kyphotic position, with sclerosed sacro iliac joints and a 'bamboo-spine' (Fig. 2.3). Involvement of the costo-vertebral joints restrict the chest expansion. In its milder forms the diagnosis depends on a history of an inflammatory type back pain, and a raised erythrocyte sedimentation rate. Sacroiliitis may not be manifest radiologically for a year or two after the onset of the illness, when radioscintigraphy with bone-seeking isotopes is more helpful in the early diagnosis (Szanto and Hagenfeldt, 1983, Rosenthall and Lisbona, 1980).

Many backache sufferers may have a sub-clinical type of ankylosing spondylitis, and the diagnosis is missed for years, if not indefinitely. It is suggested that the condition may affect two per cent of the whole population, and the mild form occur in the two sexes with equal frequency (Jayson, 1981).

There is an increased incidence of B-27 HLA antigen in ankylosing spondylitis. Jajic (1979) has reported an incidence of 42 per cent of patients with B-27 HLA antigen attending a routine back pain clinic, compared with an incidence of 7-12 per cent in the general population, but this unusually high incidence may be related to the pattern of referral.

Inflammatory changes start in the sacro iliac joints and if progressive will gradually spread cranially up the spine involving the apophyseal joints, the vertebral end plates and ligamentous attachments, until the ligaments are ossified. Hips, knees and feet may be affected. Rarely the spine will stiffen without much pain. One third of the patients develop iritis, some ulcerative colitis or Crohn's disease, and

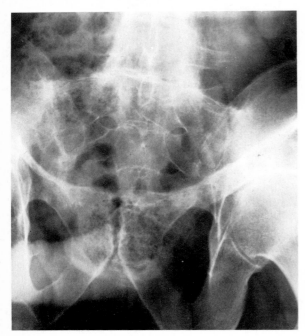

Fig. 2.3 A   A–P radiograph of a 42 year old man with an eighteen year history of ankylosing spondylitis showing sacroiliac fusion and degenerative changes of the hips.

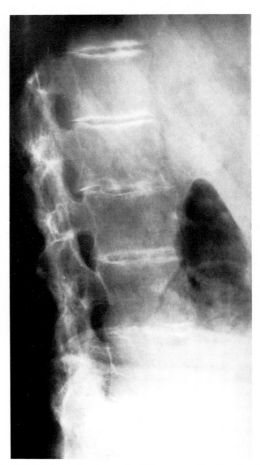

Fig. 2.3 B   Lateral radiograph of the same patient's ankylosed lumbar spine.

occasionally aortic valvular disease. These patients are most effectively treated by Rheumatologists with care to maintain a good posture, courses of anti inflammatory drugs, and mobilisation regimes.

Sacro-iliitis may follow acute salpingitis or prostatitis, and be responsible for sacro iliac pain and tenderness, and morning stiffness. Scintigraphy will be more helpful than radiography in the early diagnosis, though ultimately erosions and sclerosis develop, sometimes with complete fusion of the joint. The ESR does not correlate with the joint activity. There is a high incidence of B–27 HLA antigen. It is worth giving antibiotics for any persistent pelvic infection and sacro iliac pain (Szanto and Hagenfeldt 1979, 1983).

It is to be expected that the majority of patients consulting a rheumatologist with back pain will have an inflammatory cause, but in general this is only a small proportion of back pain sufferers. The vast majority of patients with pain in the lower back have had a mechanical disturbance and it is to the management of this problem that we are addressing this book.

REFERENCES

Allen E H, Cosgrave D, Mullard F J C 1978 The radiological changes in infections of the spine and their diagnostic value. Clinical Radiology 29: 31–40

Calin A 1979 Back pain: mechanical or inflammatory? American Family Physician 20: 97–100

Digby J M, Kersley J B 1979 Pyogenic non-tuberculous spinal infection. Journal of Bone and Joint Surgery 61–B: 47–55

Farrington M, Eykyn S J, Walker M, Warren R E 1983 Vertebral Osteomyelitis due to coccobacilli of the HB group. British Medical Journal 287: 1658–1660

Finneson B E 1973 Low Back Pain. J.B. Lippencott Co. Philadelphia and Toronto p 307.

Flood B M, Deacon P, Dickson R A 1983 Spinal disease
presenting as acute abdominal pain. British Medical Journal
287: 616–617

Freiberger R E 1960 Osteoid osteoclastoma of the spine. A cause
of backache and scoliosis in children and young adults.
Radiology 75: 232

Horne N W 1984 Problems of tuberculosis in decline. British
Medical Journal 288: 1249–1251

Jajic I 1979 The role of HLA B–27 in the diagnosis of low back
pain. Acta Orthop. Scand. 50: 411–413

Jayson M I V 1981 Back pain: the facts. Oxford University
Press. New York, Toronto

Kirwan E O'G, Hutton P A N, Pozo J L, Ransford A O 1984
Osteoid osteoma and benign osteoblastoma of the spine:
clinical presentation and treatment. Journal of Bone and
Joint Surgery 66–B: 21–26

Lichyenstein L 1975 Diseases of bones and joints. C V Mosby
Company Saint Louis, p 61

McCulloch J A, Waddell G 1978 Needle biopsy. L A and image
intensifyer control, lateral approach. British Journal of
Radiology 51: 498

Pryor J P, Castle W M, Dukes D C et al 1983 Do Beta-
Adrenoceptor blocking drugs cause retroperitoneal fibrosis?
British Medical Journal 287, 639–641

Rae P S, Waddell C and Venner R W 1984 A simple technique
for measuring lumbar spinal flexion. Journal of the Royal
College of Surgeons of Edinburgh 29: 281–284

Ratcliffe J F 1982 An evaluation of the intra-osseous arterial
anastomoses in the human vertebral body at different ages. A
microarteriographic study. Journal of Anatomy 134: 373–382

Roaf R 1980 Spinal deformities. Pitman Medical 2nd edition
p 65.

Rosenthall L, Lisbona R 1980 Role of radionuclide imaging in
benign bone and joint disease of orthopaedic interest. In:
Freeman LM Weissman HS eds, Nuclear Medicine annual
New York: Raven Press 267–301

Russell N A, Vaughan R, Morley T P 1979 Spinal epidural
infection. Le Journal Canadien Des Sciences Neurologiques
6: 325–328

Szanto E, Hangenfeldt K 1979 Sacroiliitis and salpingitis.
Quantitative 99mTc Pertechnetate in the study of sacroiliitis
in women. Scandinavian Journal of Rheumatology 8: 129

Szanto E, Hagenfeldt K 1983 Sacro-iliitis in women. A sequela
to acute salpingitis. Scandinavian Journal of Rheumatology
12: 89–92

Turek S L 1976 Orthopaedic principles and their appliances.
Pitman Medical Publishing Co. Ltd. London.

3

Structures that fail

If sufficient force is applied to any structure it will deform and fail. The spine is no exception, but the particular structures of the spine which fail depend upon the nature of the applied force, the position of the spine at the time, and the morphological variations. These differ from one individual to another and are age and sex related.

THE VERTEBRAE

A vertical compression force tends to cause an anterior wedge fracture of the vertebral bodies, T.12, L.1 and L.2 being most commonly fractured, with decreasing incidence proximally and distally (Young, 1973). The compression force necessary to fracture the vertebral bodies is inversely related to their mineral content, though it is not necessarily a linear relationship (Chapter 20). Forced flexion of the spine, such as that caused by a blow across the shoulders, will also fracture the vertebral bodies, and forced flexion and rotation will sometimes damage the posterior elements and cause neurological injury (Holdsworth, 1963).

The lumbar articular facets carry 16 to 40 per cent of the total intervertebral compressive spinal load in the erect posture (Farfan, 1973, Hakim and King, 1976, Adams and Hutton, 1980). It would not be surprising if these joints were injured at times of excessive loading.

Fracture of the apophyseal facet may be a more common source of back pain than is generally recognised (Scott, 1942, Sims-Williams et al, 1978). It may only be demonstrated on an oblique radiograph, and it must be distinguished from an accessory ossicle. We shall make the diagnosis only if it is anticipated in the patient with a short history of sudden pain following a dynamic injury. It will be supported by scintigraphy (Kuusela, 1980, Matin 1983).

In general, however, the bony structures of the young healthy spine have a considerable margin of safety when subjected to the forces of maximum lifts (Hutton and Adams, 1982). On the other hand, in the older demineralised spine microfractures of the articular facets and remodelling in response to stress are probable factors permitting gradual forward displacement of L.4 on L.5 in degenerative spondylolisthesis (Newman, 1963).

Microfractures also accompany disruption of the vertebral end plate by disc herniation, and the development of Schmorl's nodes (Hilton, 1980), and some degree of skeletal failure results in the 'cod-fish' appearance of demineralised vertebrae (Fig. 20.3).

'THE INTERVERTEBRAL DISC

1. Mechanism of failure

The disc fails when the nucleus pulposus extrudes either through a fissure in the annulus or as a Schmorl's node through the vertebral end-plate posteriorly, centrally or anteriorly. The force necessary to produce this failure is dependant both upon individual anatomical variations, and age. For example, a compression force which will produce a wedge fracture in the middle aged adult will produce vertical extrusion of disc nucleus through the end plate in an adolescent or young healthy adult.

There is an age related tendency to disc failure, disc symptoms presenting for the first time most frequently in the fourth decade. Either the annulus is

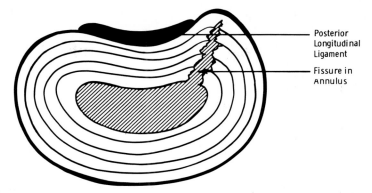

Fig. 3.1 Diagram to show the common site of an annular fissure at the site of the maximum convexity, just lateral to the posterior longitudinal ligament.

more resilient in the young, or there are protecting mechanisms resisting failure. There are certainly progressive microscopic and biochemical changes in the nucleus and annulus. Urban and Maroudas (1980) have reviewed the chemistry of the intervertebral disc showing that there is a progressive fall in water content of the nucleus with increased collagen, lower glycosaminoglycan levels, breakdown of the proteoglycans and a fall in the fixed charge density. The nucleus becomes less homogenous with age, more inspissated with loss of its basic hydrostatic properties (Harris and Macnab, 1954). Perhaps a fall in annular resilience is balanced by a change in the nucleus making it less vulnerable to prolapse, with greatest risk in middle life.

When an annular tear occurs, it generally is posteriorly, just lateral to the posterior longitudinal ligament (Fig. 3.1) where the non-circular geometry of the disc concentrates stress at the site of maximum convexity (Farfan, 1973, Hickey and Hukins, 1980). The fissure can develop gradually, from the inner to the outer layers of the annulus, or suddenly disrupt all the layers with a nuclear herniation. The many layers of obliquely placed annular fibres are so arranged that each adjacent layer is orientated in an opposite direction, producing a 'radial ply' effect (Fig. 3.2). By this arrangement intact annular fibres will contain the nucleus even when it is subjected to a vertical compression force that would normally fracture a vertebra. If there is already an annular fissure (either a congenital weakness (Dixon 1973) or from previous trauma), the resilience of the disc is reduced, and the remaining peripheral annular fibres

can be disrupted now, by either a rotational or a vertical compression force.

Opinions differ, in the type of force required to tear the annulus. Hickey and Hukins (1980) suggest that rotation is important whilst Adams and Hutton (1981, 1982) believe that compression of the flexed spine is particularly damaging.

It is probably not axial compression, however, but compression in flexion or torsion that is likely to constitute the first injury to an intact annulus (Hickey and Hukins, 1980). By analogy with behaviour of tendon, it has been estimated that approximately four degrees of torsion will stretch beyond the elastic limit those layers of annular fibres which are orientated against the torsion, and that further torsion or flexion will tear them (Klein et al, 1982). Even four degrees is probably in excess of the torsion permitted by the

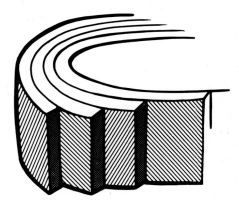

Fig. 3.2 Diagram to show that the layers of the annulus have their fibres orientated obliquely in alternate directions, to produce a radial ply effect.

restraining apophyseal joints at L.4/5 and at L.5/Sl, unless the spine is first flexed to disengage these joints. Rotation of a flexed spine is probably actively resisted by reflex muscle action, but a superadded fall or unexpected strain may overcome that protective reflex and produce sufficient torsion to damage a healthy annulus. This mechanism of disc injury fits both the known facts of the functional anatomy of the spine, and also the clinical explanation of the first injury, often recounted by patients — a fall or an unexpected strain causing the patient to twist whilst in the stooping position.

2. Disc resilience

We have no evidence to date that disc resilience bears any relation to spinal stress in the developing years, though it might be expected. In other anatomical sites, function and form go hand in hand, and probably hard work produces a strong annulus. Kelsey (1975) showed that there was a greater incidence of herniated discs in sedentary workers: perhaps 'further education' is responsible for many a weak back and subsequent disc excision. Our own studies suggest that miners have a lesser incidence of acute disc prolapse and herniation, though they are much more prone to the back pain syndromes associated with degenerative change (root entrapment and neurogenic claudication).

3. Disc nutrition

The lumbar intervertebral discs are the largest avascular structures in the body. Their resilience to withstand injury depends on adequate nutrition, but when is nutrition inadequate? It probably depends on a satisfactory capillary bed in the vertebral body adjacent to the cartilaginous end plate. Impairment of this capillary bed from bony sclerosis, from raised intraosseous venous pressure or from the age-related changes in intraosseous arterial anatomy (Ratcliffe, 1982), can affect disc nutrition, and may be responsible for some of the progressive biochemical changes in the disc. The epidemiological studies of Frymoyer and his colleagues (1983) have shown that back pain is more frequent in smokers and those individuals whose spines are subjected to high frequency vibrations. They postulate that small changes in the capillary bed from toxic agents or from vibration may significantly affect disc nutrition.

The avascular disc depends on the passage of fluid into the collagen matrix for its nutrition. Solutes pass rapidly into the disc by diffusion but large molecules are slow to pass through the fine proteoglycan meshwork. Diurnal changes in fluid volume is considerable and probably aids nutrition (Adams and Hutton, 1983). Disc hydration depends upon a balance between the osmotic pressure within the disc, and the hydrostatic pressure forcing fluid out of the disc. The volume increases as the hydrostatic pressure is reduced by recumbency, and then the osmotic pressure is largely unopposed. Conversely, the vertical posture increases the hydrostatic pressure diminishing the fluid volume. Much of the diurnal change in standing height is due to change in the disc's fluid volume. This can amount to 2 cm during the day and it fluctuates fairly quickly with change of posture (Reilly et al, 1984, Eklund and Corlett, 1984). Postural change, and rest between periods of strenuous work affects fluid flow and is probably beneficial to disc nutrition.

There is much interest in the chemistry of the disc in disease. The identification of enzymes is providing a better understanding of the degradation process but we are still uncertain whether injury alters disc nutrition and hence its chemistry, or whether altered nutrition affects the biochemistry of the disc making it vulnerable to injury.

4. The 'motor segment'

It is too easy to think of the disc as an isolated structure, and fail to recognise it as part of a 'motor segment' (Lewin et al, 1962, Schmorl and Junghanns, 1971), incorporating the apophyseal joints in a three-joint system. Disruption of a disc must result in disturbed function of the three joint system, if not at the time of the disc failure, then in subsequent years.

Osteophytes result from spinal stress (though are not necessarily associated with spinal symptoms). Macnab (1971, 1977) differentiated between claw and traction spurs. Claw type osteophytes develop at the edge of the vertebral body margin around the annulus and sometimes meet and fuse the two vertebrae together (Fig. 3.3). They are commonly seen on the convex side of a scoliosis, and may or may not be

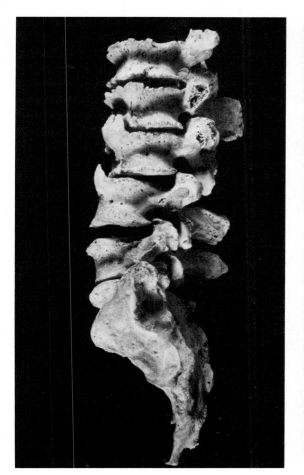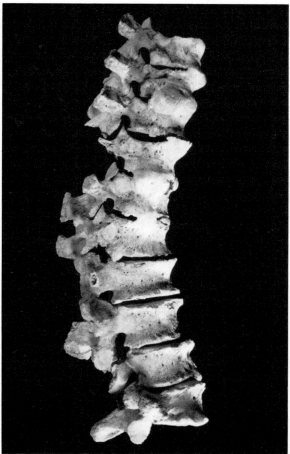

Fig. 3.3 a) 'Claw type' osteophytic spurs from the edge of the vertebral body; b) Sometimes these osteophytes produce an inter-body fusion.

associated with disc degeneration. Traction spurs develop a few millimeters from the upper and lower borders of the vertebral bodies (Fig. 3.4) and grow into the attachment of the anterior longitudinal ligament and annular fibres. They are generally accepted as a sign of 'instability' (Harris and Macnab, 1954), (Chapter 15), and the majority are associated with disc degeneration (Quinnell and Stockdale, 1982). In practice, there is a spectrum of osteophytes from claw to traction spurs, the classification of a particular osteophyte depending on the particular radiological projection (Macnab, 1971). The two particular types may both be related to spinal stress, but from forces in different planes, and may be a sign of protection rather than failure.

If osteophytes are not an invariable sign of disc

failure, nevertheless disc failure is followed by osteophyte formation within a decade, not only by lipping of the anterior or antero-lateral margins of the vertebral bodies, but sometimes posteriorly by vertebral bar formation, and generally by osteophytes at the margins of the apophyseal joints (Vernon-Roberts, 1980).

SPINAL LIGAMENTS

Isolated disruption of ligaments may occasionally occur as a result of spinal stress but it is a difficult diagnosis to prove, except in the combined bony ligamentous injury of unstable fracture and fracture-

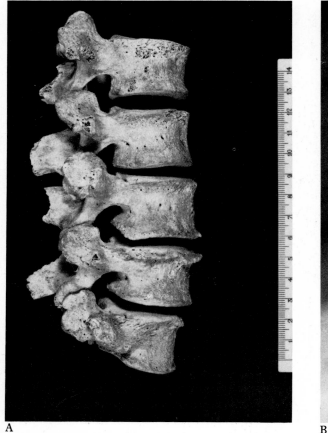
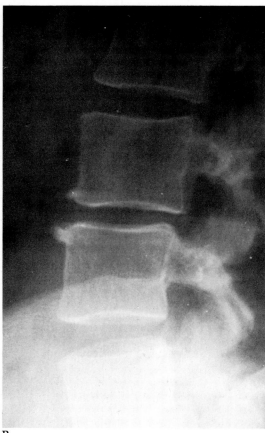

A   B

Fig. 3.4   A) Five Romano-British lumbar vertebrae showing traction spurs on the adjacent margins of L3/4 vertebral bodies;
B) Radiograph of a patient with traction spurs at L3/4 level, reduction of disc space and signs of rotational instability.

dislocation of the spine (Nicoll, 1949). Adams and Hutton (1982) suspect that interspinous ligament failure may be the pre-cursor of disc injury, by permitting an unacceptable degree of segmental flexion, subsequently overloading the disc. Disruption of the interspinous and supraspinous ligaments may also precede degenerative spondylolisthesis (Newman, 1963).

The orientation of the fibres of the interspinous ligament are certainly very interesting from a functional aspect, passing obliquely from the spinous process above to be attached more anteriorly to the spinous process below (Heylings, 1978, 1980). This does permit a controlled arc of forward flexion of the adjacent vertebrae (whilst a vertical orientation would permit no flexion at all). Disruption would certainly interfere with smooth restrained forward flexion and extension increasing the demands on other restraining structures.

The complex anatomical arrangement of the lumbar fascia (Fig. 3.5) provides attachments between the spinous processes and supra spinous ligaments in the mid line, through the posterior layer of the fascia, and attachments to the transverse processes through the middle and anterior layers on the posterior and anterior surfaces of the quadratus lumborum. These three layers combine to form attachments laterally to the three layers of the abdominal muscles, the latissimus dorsi and the glutei. Thus, together, the layers of the lumbar fascia form a dynamic structure rather than a static rigid mechanism of stability. There is a concept that this is reinforced by the two

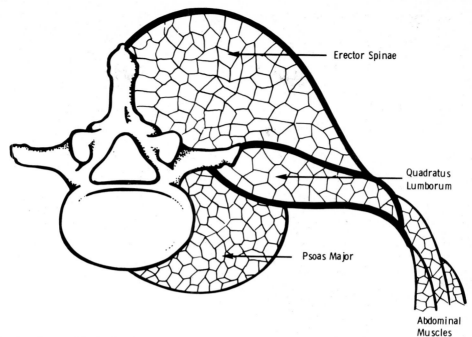

Fig. 3.5 The three layers of the lumbar fascia attached to the spinous and transverse processes of the lumbar vertebrae, which through the abdominal and para spinal muscles, assist stability.

leaves of the supraspinous ligament separated by fatty tissue and the cruciate architecture of the posterior layer of lumbar fascia (Fig. 3.6). Lateral tension through the lumbar fascia separates these two leaves of the supraspinous ligament increasing tension and restraining separation of the spinous processes. Thus, with the paraspinal muscles, the ligamentous structures form an active dynamic restraining unit to

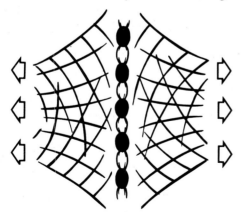

Fig. 3.6 Diagram to show how the posterior layer of the lumbar fascia is attached to the lumbar spinous processes and the two leaves of the supraspinous ligament. Contraction of the abdominal muscles will restrain spinal flexion.

protect the spine from unguarded flexion (Bogduk and MacIntosh, 1984). It is reasonable to assume that damage to the ligamentous complex will predispose the spine to mechanical failure. If the transverse processes can be avulsed by contusion, probably the lumbar fascia can be disrupted by similar forces also. The concept of dynamic ligamentous support is a salutary reminder to the surgeon not to interfere unnecessarily with these structures, either by excision, promoting scar tissue or by denervating sections of the muscle.

The pregnancy hormone relaxin has been shown to permit increased spinal mobility in addition to pelvic laxity (Calguneri et al, 1982). The female spine is particularly vulnerable to injury in pregnancy, and the laxity of ligaments may be a responsible factor.

Disruption of the lumbar fascia above the posterior iliac crest can result in a painful hernia of retroperitoneal fat, sometimes becoming gangrenous and requiring excision and repair (Light, 1983).

SPINAL MUSCLES

Muscle rupture, disruption at a musculo-tendinous junction, or avulsion of ligamentous attachments are probably just as common in the spine as in the limbs, but because of the inaccessibility of spinal structures, isolated muscle injury is less easily diagnosed. It may be suspected, however, in a young athlete or an individual suddenly experiencing unusually high stress, whose tenderness is localised away from the mid line. Discomfort is experienced when the muscle involved is stretched or movement is resisted. For instance, tenderness above the posterior iliac crest in a young footballer, with pain extending into the buttock, whose pain is aggravated by spinal flexion and adduction of the hip, or resisted spinal extension or resisted adduction of the hip, probably is a musculo-tendinous injury rather than a mechanical disturbance of the lumbar spine. A cortisone injection and ultrasound therapy is more likely to help than enforced rest. It is difficult to refute those who maintain that muscle sprains and ligamentous strains are the commonest cause of low back pain. There are no absolute diagnostic criteria, and the occasional cure by injection does not convince the sceptic.

The security of the spine depends greatly upon the protective response of the para spinal and abdominal muscles to posture and movement (Nachemson, 1966, Schultz et al, 1982). The involuntary reflex balance of the supporting muscles plays a large part in preventing failure of other spinal structures. Too frequently we are told by our patients that their first spinal injury occurred in an unguarded moment, perhaps when slipping on a floor, dropping suddenly down a step, or having to support a weight when a colleague fell. Nurses not infrequently injure their backs when lifting an unco-operative patient who makes an unexpected movement. Stress applied suddenly, before the muscle response is able to protect the spine, is probably a common cause of failure and disc injury.

The abdominal muscles play an important part in supporting the spine (Farfan, 1973, Davis and Stubbs, 1976) partly by producing sufficient intra-abdominal pressure to splint the anterior and lateral aspects of the vertebral column, partly by their attachments to the lumbar fascia, and partly as a load carrier. Davis, using a pressure transducer in the form of a swallowed pill, has postulated a good correlation between intra abdominal pressure and mechanical stress on the spine. The role of the hip extensors which play a major part in the early component of lifting, has been largely ignored.

There is a relationship between the static and dynamic spinal muscle strength, and the ability to lift without injury (Chaffin et al, 1978). Patients with low back pain do have significantly lower strength and greater fatigability of trunk muscles than healthy controls even when the history of back pain is short (Suzuki and Endo, 1983), but it is not certain whether this is cause or effect.

The frequency of muscle injury as a source of back pain is debatable, but there is no doubt that the abdominal and spinal muscles are important components of spinal protection and that their strength should meet the tasks required of the spine.

THE PROTECTIVE ROLE OF THE APOPHYSEAL JOINTS

The annulus is vulnerable to excessive rotational strain, but is protected by the configuration of the apophyseal joints, by the splinting effects of the spinal ligaments and lumbar fascia, by the dynamic action of the trunk and abdominal muscles, and by the intra-abdominal pressure. It is in an unguarded moment such as a stumble or a fall that the mechanism may fail, and this is more likely to occur if the lumbar spine is in the flexed position at the time of the injury than in extension.

When the lumbar spine is extended, the apophyseal joints are in the 'close packed' position, with the male and female surfaces of the joints fitting point-for-point (MacConaill, 1950). In flexion the joints are in 'loose pack' with incongruity of the two surfaces, because the male surface has a smaller curvature than the female, and the two surfaces come into contact only at one point. It is in this loose-packed position, in flexion, that the musculo-ligamentous complex actively protects against excessive rotation, and should it fail, the annulus is prone to tear. In the close packed position, in full extension, the apophyseal joints provide a fail-safe mechanism, hence the advice that one should lift with a lordotic lumbar spine.

Professional weight lifters have found that they achieve better results in this posture (Fig. 3.7), perhaps because in the close packed position the posterior column of the spine bears greater proportion of the load, up to 40 per cent of the total vertebral compressive spinal load.

Myeloelectric activity of the trunk and abdominal

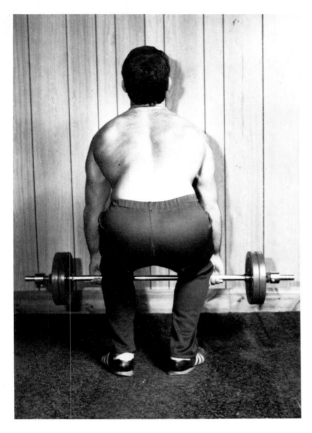

muscles is less with the spine in the upright position, when twisting and lateral flexing, than when in the flexed position (Schultz et al, 1982). Both apophyseal joints are in close-pack in the upright posture, one will be close packed when twisting and in lateral flexion; in the loose-packed position, flexion is maintained at the expense of increased muscle activity. One may argue that if it is essential to lift by bending forwards, the spine should be lordotic. If flexed there is greater expenditure of energy and the disc is vulnerable to an accidental twisting injury.

Any spinal structure can fail, be it muscle, ligament, bone or joint, but in practice the intervertebral disc is the main problem. Other structures of the motor segment are involved both in the mechanism of disc injury and in the subsequent pathological process, but the disc should be central in our thinking about back pain.

Fig. 3.7 The lordotic spine of the professional weightlifter.

REFERENCES

Adams M A, Hutton W C 1980 The effect of posture on the role of the apophyseal joints in resisting intervertebral compressive forces. Journal of Bone and Joint Surgery 62B: 358

Adams M A, Hutton W C 1981 The relevance of torsion to the mechanical derangement of the lumbar spine. Spine 6: 241–248

Adams M A and Hutton W C 1982 Prolapsed intervertebral disc — a hyperflexion injury. Spine 7: 184–191

Adams M A and Hutton W C 1983 The effect of posture on the fluid content of lumbar intervertebral discs, Spine 8: 665–671

Bogduk N and MacIntosh J E 1984 The applied anatomy of the thoraco-lumbar fascia. Spine 9: 164–170

Calguneri M, Bird H A, Wright V 1982. Changes in joint laxity occurring during pregnancy. Annals of the Rheumatic Diseases 41: 126–128

Chaffin D B, Herrin G D, Keyserling W M 1978 Pre-employment strength testing: an updated position. Journal of Occupational Medicine 20: 403

Davis P R, Stubbs D A 1976 A method of establishing safe handling forces in working situations. Symposium on safety in manual materials handling at Suny, Buffalo, organised by National Institute of Occupational Safety and Health

Dixon A St. J 1973 Progress and Problems in Back Pain Research. Rheumatology and Rehabilitation 12, 165–175

Eklund J A and Corlett E N 1984 Shrinkage as a measure of the effect of load on the spine. Spine (in press)

Farfan H F 1973 The mechanical disorders of the lower back. Philadelphia, Lea and Febiger

Frymoyer J W, Pope M H, Clements J H, Wilder D G, MacPhearson B, Ashikaga T 1983. Risk factors in low back pain. Journal of Bone and Joint Surgery 65-A: 213–218

Hakim N S, King A I 1976 Static and dynamic articular facet loads. Proc. 20th Stapp Car Crash Conf 609

Harris R I, Macnab I 1954 Structural changes in degeneration of the lumbar intervertebral disc: their relationship to low back pain and sciatica. Journal of Bone and Joint Surgery 36-B: 304–322

Heylings D J A 1978 Supraspinous and interspinous ligaments of the human lumbar spine. Journal of Anatomy 125: 127–131

Heylings D J A 1980 Supraspinous and interspinous ligaments in dog, cat and baboon. Journal of Anatomy 130: 223–228

Hickey D S, Hukins D W L 1980 Spine 5: 106

Hilton R C 1980 Systematic studies of spinal mobility and Schmorl's nodes. The Lumbar Spine and Back Pain. Ed. Jayson. 2nd Edn. The Pitman Press Bath.

Holdsworth F W 1963 Fractures, dislocations and fracture-dislocations of the spine. Journal of Bone and Joint Surgery 45-B: 6–20

Hutton W C and Adams M A 1982 Can the lumbar spine be crushed in heavy lifting? Spine 7: 586–590

Kelsey J L 1975 An epidemiological study of acute herniated lumbar intervertebral discs. Rheumatology and Rehabilitation 14: 144–159

Klein J A, Hickey D S, Hukins D W L 1982 Computer graphics illustration of the operation of the intervertebral disc. Engineering in Medicine 11: 11–15

Kuusela T V 1980 Stress fracture. A radionuclide, roentgenological and clinical study of Finnish conscripts. Thesis. The department of Roentgenology, University of Oulu, Finland

Lewin T, Moffett B, Viidik A 1962 The morphology of the lumbar synovial intervertebral joints. Acta Morphologica Neerlando-Scandinavica, Vol. 4: 229–319

Light H G 1983 Hernia of the inferior lumbar space. A cause of back pain. Arch. Surg. 118: 1077–80

MacConaill M A 1950 The movements of bones and joints. Journal of Bone and Joint Surgery, 32–B: 244–252

Macnab I 1971 The traction spur. Journal of Bone and Joint Surgery 53–A: 663–670

Macnab I 1977 Backache. Baltimore: Williams and Wilkins Co.

Matin P 1983 Bone scintigraphy in the diagnosis and management of traumatic injury. Seminar of Nuclear Medicine 13: 104–122

Nachemson A 1966 Electromyographic studies on the vertebral portion of the psoas muscle. Acta Orthop Scandanav 37: 177–190

Newman P H 1963 The Etiology of Spondylolisthesis. Journal of Bone and Joint Surgery 45–B: 39–59

Nicoll E A 1949 Fractures of the dorso-lumbar spine. Journal of Bone and Joint Surgery 31–B: 376–394

Quinnell R C, Stockdale H R 1982 The significance of osteophytes on the lumbar vertebral bodies in relation to discographic findings. Clinical Radiology 23: 197–203

Ratcliffe J F 1982 An evaluation of the intra-osseous arterial anastomoses in the human vertebral body at different ages. A microarteriographic study. Journal of Anatomy 134: 373–382

Reilly T, Tyrrell A R and Troup J D G 1984 Circadian variation in human stature. Chronobiology Int. Journal (in press)

Schmorl G, Junghanns H 1971 The human spine in health and disease. 2nd American Edition. New York Grune and Strathon

Schultz A B, Andersson G B J, Haderspeck K, Ortengren R, Nordin M, Bjork R 1982 Analysis and measurement of lumbar trunk loads in tasks involving bends and twists. Journal of Biomechanics 15: 669–675

Scott W G 1942 Low back pain resulting from arthritis and subluxations of the apophyseal joints and fractures of the articular facets of the lumbar spine. American Journal of Bone and Joint Surgery 48: 491–509

Sims-Williams H, Jayson M I V, Young S M S, Baddeley H, Collins E 1978 Controlled trial of mobilisation and manipulation for patients with low back pain in general practice. British Medical Journal 2, 1338–1340

Suzuki N, Endo S 1983 A quantitative study of trunk muscle strength and fatigability in the low back pain syndrome. Spine 8: 59–74

Urban J and Maroudas A 1980 The chemistry of the intervertebral disc in relation to its physiological function and requirements. Clinics in Rheumatic Diseases 6 (1) 51–75

Vernon-Roberts B 1980 The Lumbar Spine and Back Pain, P. 108. Jayson M I V ed. Pitman Medical Ltd

Young M H 1973 Long term consequences of stable fractures of the thoracic and lumbar vertebral bodies. Journal of Bone and Joint Surgery 55–B: 295–300

4

The pain source

Pain is difficult to define, but can be considered as an unpleasant abnormal experience. It generally has a source, and when investigating a patient with back pain, we endeavour to find often without success, that source.

The majority of tissues in the spine with the exception of the bone have been shown to contain nerve endings which could be pain receptors (Wyke, 1980). They have been identified in the capsule of the apophyseal joints, the posterior longitudinal ligament, the interspinous ligament, the ligamentum flavum, the dura, especially the anterior surface, the epidural adipose tissue, the vertebral periosteum, the walls of the arterioles and veins, the vessels of the paravertebral muscles and the annulus of the disc where it merges with the posterior longitudinal ligament contains free nerve endings (Yoshizawa et al, 1980, Bogduk et al, 1981). Any of these tissues are possible originators of pain when injury produces either a mechanical stimulus or chemical alteration of the interstitial fluid.

It is possible, however, that some of these nerve endings are not pain receptors. It is difficult to conceive that they are present in such abundance merely to sound an alarm at the first hint of injury. Perhaps for the majority of the time they serve other functions, and only at a threshold do they produce pain. Any nerve receptor, if stimulated above a threshold, may become a source of pain. Too intense a light or loud a sound produces pain. A temperature too hot or cold is painful. Too great a pressure on the skin, or tension on a joint capsule may change the normal nerve function to pain. In the spine, structures well endowed with free nerve endings may also be a pain source if the stimulus is sufficiently intense. Unfortunately we cannot yet identify from the information available which structure is actually responsible for the experienced pain.

That is not to say we cannot suggest probabilities of the source of pain in certain back pain syndromes, nor suggest why pain is absent when there is apparent structural failure in the spine. The fact that a structure fails does not mean that it is the source of pain. Mechanical stress to the spine may produce segmental failure, with disc degeneration, disc space narrowing, and osteophyte formation in a subject who has never experienced back pain. Many elderly women have degenerative spondylolisthesis with forward displacement of the body of L.4 on L.5 without symptoms. It is perhaps not surprising that free nerve endings have not been recorded in disc nucleus, bone or cartilage, for the most degenerate spines can be symptomless.

THE APOPHYSEAL JOINTS

The posterior joints must be considered in association with disc space degeneration. They are invariably degenerate if the associated disc space is narrowed. Many believe that the apophyseal joints are a frequent source of back pain, but why can they be degenerate and symptom free? Perhaps it is for the same reason that the terminal interphalangeal joints of the hands can be arthritic yet painless, or the toe joints deformed and degenerate without pain. The apophyseal joints are presumably painful if the capsule is stretched with synovial swelling, or by excessive excursion, or if there is increased pressure in the subchondral vessels, but degenerative change alone is not necessarily painful.

Some structures in the spine can presumably fail

and produce pain for a short period, until healing occurs. For example, a compression fracture of a vertebral body becomes painless after a few weeks in 26 per cent of patients (Young, 1973). One would expect fractures of apophyseal joints, microfractures, stress fractures, and disc extrusion through a vertebral end plate to produce only temporary pain, unless other structures are affected. Likewise, ligamentous or muscular injuries producing self-limiting back pain should not be a chronic problem. The majority of patients with back pain, especially those with a chronic problem, probably have an alternative pain source.

STRUCTURES RESTRAINING SHEAR

The thickened capsule and ligaments of an osteoarthritic hip can cause pain when stretched, and it is not unreasonable to assume that the ligamentous and capsular structures of the spine which restrain shearing forces are likewise a source of pain. They are well endowed with free nerve endings. Injection of hypertonic saline stretching the capsule of the apophyseal joints will produce referred pain to the ipsilateral side of the lower back, the buttock and even into the posterior thigh (McCall et al, 1979).

The maximum shearing forces are at L.5/S.1, but are well resisted by the strong ilio-lumbar and lumbo-sacral ligament, the disc and the coronally orientated apophyseal joint. Lysis of the pars interarticularis negates the effect of the posterior joints, but the other supporting structures are usually adequate. These are probably a source of pain should they fail. Patients with isthmic spondylolisthesis who attend hospital commonly complain of pain in the back referred into the buttocks and posterior thighs. This would seem to be associated with shearing forces, being worse when standing and shopping, and is generally relieved by lying down. A spinal fusion abolishing the effects of shear invariably resolves the problem (Attenborough and Reynolds, 1975).

The orientation of the facets at L.4/5, the weaker ligaments and the larger disc space means that shear, though less powerful at this level, is less effectively resisted. This is the commonest site for degenerative spondylolisthesis.

It is not unreasonable to suggest that structures which restrain shear can be a source of chronic backache when there is mechanical failure of the spine.

PAIN SENSITIVE STRUCTURES WITHIN THE VERTEBRAL CANAL

The dura

There are few nerve fibres in the posterior dura, and penetration by needle in the process of radiculography is seldom painful. The anterior dura, however, is richly supplied with nerve fibres and some believe this is an important pain source (Cyriax, 1978). There is much to support this concept. It can explain the relief obtained by epidural injection of local anaesthetic in the presence of disc protrusion; why subjects with a narrow vertebral canal are more prone to disc symptoms in acute prolapse; and also why segmental instability from chronic disc degeneration can be painful. It can explain the pain and limitation of lumbar extension if there is vertebral displacement, and a narrow canal (Fig. 4.1).

The nerve roots, ganglia and spinal nerve

The true spinal nerve at the lower lumbar levels is only a short segment close to the intervertebral foramina; the greatest part of the length of the nerve in the vertebral canal is composed of ventral and dorsal spinal roots with the dorsal root ganglia, the pre-ganglionic segment (Fig. 4.2). These structures are unquestionably vulnerable to mechanical disturbance within the vertebral canal, the degree depending to some extent on the variable anatomy of the nerve roots and their attachments.

Root excursion is limited proximally by dural fixation, and distally by root attachment at the intervertebral foramen. Proximally the dura is loosely attached by either multiple bands or a solid mid line septum to the posterior longitudinal ligament just proximal to the L.4/5 and L.5/S.1 disc and also by more lateral attachments (Spencer et al, 1983). The distal attachment of the root to the intervertebral foramen is relatively firm, permitting only slight distal migration of the root when traction is applied to the spinal nerve. The root is thus partly insulated from the effects of a distal traction force.

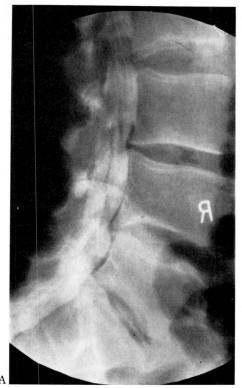
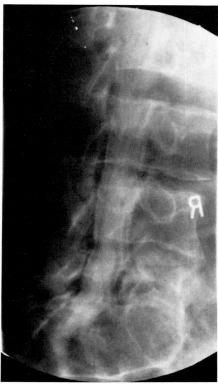

A

B

Fig. 4.1 A myelogram of a 54 year old miner with pain in the lower back radiating to the outer hips, aggravated by extension. A, Lateral view showing posterior displacement of L.4 on L.5 indenting the tight dural sac. It is easily understood that extension could produce anterior dural pain.
B, Oblique view showing posterior dural compression from the lamina of L.5.

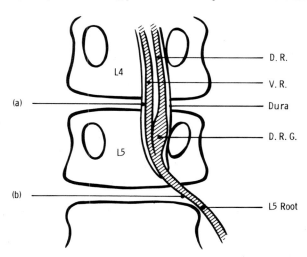

Fig. 4.2 Diagram to show L.5 dorsal and ventral roots, ganglion and spinal nerve. The roots are vulnerable from an L.4/5 disc lesion in the central canal (a), and the spinal nerve from a lateral L.5/S.1 disc lesion in the root canal (b). The ganglion may be affected at either level depending on its variable position.

Spencer and his colleagues described a further ligamentous band from the sheath of the extra dural nerve root to the inferior pedicle of the respective foramen. The variable degree of root fixation will affect the extent to which the root is tented over a disc protrusion, and may explain root symptoms in those patients with a small disc lesion and a spacious canal.

In addition, tension in the attachment of the dura to the posterior longitudinal ligament may produce those symptoms observed by Smyth and Wright (1958), who attached silk threads to the posterior longitudinal ligament and the vertebral periosteum during spinal surgery. Subsequent traction produced unilateral low back pain radiating into the ipsilateral buttock and thigh.

Root fixation is also affected by anatomical anomalies of the roots. Kadish and Simmons (1984) described anastomoses between rootlets, anomalous origins of roots, extradural anastomoses and divisions in 14 per cent of specimens examined, and these will influence root excursion.

We know little about the importance of the sinu vertebral nerve as it returns from the post ganglionic segment of the spinal nerve into the root canal. It may at times, with the nerve roots, be a pain source.

Nerve conduction can be stimulated, enhanced, altered, with or without affecting the axon transport system. The mechanical factors responsible are generally thought to be two distinct types, from disc protrusion or from bony/soft tissue degenerative changes. (A) Disc protrusion can be acute or chronic, and in the majority of instances the lesion affects the ventral and or dorsal roots in the central canal. Occasionally a lateral disc affects the lumbar root in the root canal. (B) By contrast, bony encroachment into the root canal from the apophyseal joints, from the margins of the vertebral bodies, from thickened ligamentous structures, perhaps a combination of these with unnatural segmental movement produces root involvement with a different pattern of symptoms. The post ganglionic spinal nerve is vulnerable at this level, less commonly the ganglia and the pre ganglionic nerve and roots. Occasionally the roots may be involved more proximally by the degenerative change of a prominent vertebral bar in the central canal, especially in the presence of vertebral displacement or unnatural movement.

The two types of lesion, i.e. the acute disc and the chronic degenerative process, can both affect the roots, ganglia and spinal nerve, but generally at different sites. The chronicity of the lesion, and more particularly the site, may explain the different character of pain and the different signs in patients who have the same root involvement (Leyshon et al, 1980).

The anatomy of the axons between the cord and the ganglia is unique, with the cell body of the ganglia at some distance from the synapse in the posterior horn of the cord. Rydevik (1982) has shown that this section of the dorsal root is more sensitive to ischaemia than the ventral root, perhaps explaining why a disc protrusion can produce pain and sensory loss without muscle weakness. The closer the lesion is to the ganglion, the more likely it is to cause permanent damage to the cell in the dorsal root ganglion.

Experimental compression of a nerve root will produce variable changes related to the degree of pressure. At 30 mm Hg intraneural oedema develops affecting nerve function. 50 mm Hg affects axoplasmic transport. A high pressure of 200 mm Hg such as could develop from a massive disc prolapse compressing a root against a lamina or adjacent ligamentum flavum, will deform the nerve tissue, the most significant damage occurring at the edge of the compression.

There are thus many factors that will affect the response of neural tissue to mechanical injury. The site of the compression, its degree, its duration, its nature whether soft or bony hard, the diameter of the fibre and the dynamic factors of root excursion, with irritative, inflammatory and biochemical changes. We have much to learn about lumbar root pain, but there is no question that the root and ganglion are a significant pain source.

It is possible that not only the root, but the peripheral nerve itself, becomes a pain source. The axonal protein transport may be affected at a spinal level by mechanical disturbance and make the peripheral nerve itself vulnerable to compression and irritation. This would make sense of several clinical observations. A patient with bony entrapment of the nerve root in the root canal, not uncommonly states that the root pain is precipitated by sitting on a hard surface, and it is relieved by shifting their position. The sciatic nerve in the buttock is sensitive to direct pressure producing pain from a peripheral source. Likewise some patients with bony entrapment of the root in the root canal have their most severe pain in the outer shin and dorsum of the foot. Digital compression of the lateral popliteal nerve at the neck of the fibula is acutely tender. Surgical decompression at this level often relieves the discomfort below the knee. The bowstring sign with pain behind the knee when palpating the stretched popliteal nerve, when straight leg raising is limited, is the same phenomenon. A spinal lesion may produce abnormal axonal chemistry with a pain source in the peripheral nerve itself.

One may also speculate about the source of pain when a patient describes the peripheral spread of sciatic pain, first in the buttock, then the thigh, and subsequently the calf, ankle and foot. The original pain source was at the spinal level say from a disc protrusion affecting the nerve root or ganglion, but how significant is the axon transport system of protein at 410 millimeters per day? Is the pathology only at spinal level, or is the peripheral nerve itself becoming the source of pain by its altered chemistry?

Not infrequently a patient who has had previous episodes of disc symptoms with root pain, will have a recurrence of symptoms when convalescing from a 'flu-like' illness. This could be a mechanical phenomenon, with injury to a disc, bulging from the reduced hydrostatic pressure of a few day's recumbency, and unsupported by atrophied muscles. One must question, however, whether the root ganglion could be affected by viraemia, if previously bruised from a disc prolapse. Certainly the virus of herpes latent within spinal ganglia, can be periodically activated (Caplan et al, 1977, Warren et al, 1978).

Cerebrospinal fluid

The function of the cerebrospinal fluid surrounding the cauda equina is still ill-understood. It buffers the roots and ganglia against physical stress, much as the foetus is protected by liquor. It probably has an insulting effect on nerve conduction, and may be a source of nutrition and remover of nerve metabolites. We do not know what influence a reduced volume of cerebrospinal fluid has on the cauda equina in such syndromes as neurogenic claudication, nor on its elimination from the dural sheath of a root compressed by a disc protrusion — 'the cut off sign' commonly seen on radiculography (Fig. 4.3). The absence of cerebrospinal fluid in adhesive arachnoiditis may have symptomatic importance. Its influence on nerve function may be highly significant.

The blood supply

Nerve tissue is particularly vulnerable to ischaemia. The function of the ganglia and roots may be adversely affected by local ischaemia from compression, or secondarily from vascular insufficiency. Domminisse (1975) has described the abundant arterial supply to each lumbar nerve root, with the smallest radicular capillaries no larger than five microns and the posterior root ganglion having a particularly rich concentration. The supply is abundant presumably because it is necessary, and if it becomes deficient from mechanical compression,

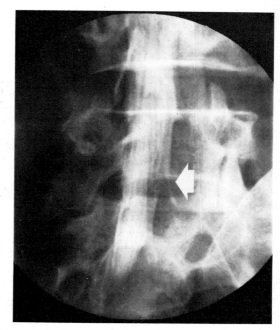

Fig. 4.3 Radiculogram of a 32 year old woman with left S.1 root pain, reduced straight leg raising, and altered sensation of the outer foot. The metrizamide does not enter the left S.1 root dural sac, the 'cut off' sign of disc protrusion.

scarring or traction, it probably affects nerve function.

The proximal third of the roots of the cauda equina are supplied by the spinal arteries from above, anastomosing with the radicular arteries at the junction of the upper and middle thirds. This crescenteric watershed is relatively vulnerable to ischaemia when the radicular supply is deficient.

The relationship between the intraosseous lumbar arterial supply and the radicular arteries has not been established, but it would not be surprising if in certain pathological conditions, it became significant. The upper four lumbar arteries are posterior branches of the abdominal aorta arising opposite the bodies of the upper four lumbar vertebra. A fifth pair usually arises from the ilio-lumbar artery, but occasionally from the median sacral. These arteries soon divide and run laterally and backwards on the bodies of the lumbar vertebrae, supplying intraosseous branches to the vertebral bodies, then a radicular branch through the intervertebral foramen before further branches supply the muscles of the back and the abdominal wall. The intraosseous arteries are particularly interesting showing a marked coiling, which increases

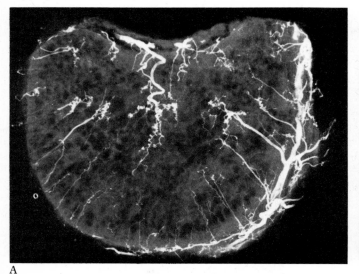
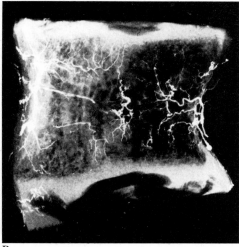

A   B

Fig. 4.4   A, coronal section of lumbar vertebral body showing the coiling of the intra osseous branches of the lumbar arteries. B, sagittal section of lumbar vertabral body. (With kind permission of Dr Ratcliffe.)

with age (Fig. 4.4). Ratcliffe (1980, 1981, 1982) described these coils, but their function is not understood. It is tempting to suggest that they may produce a resistance to arterial flow, acting as a hydrostatic dampener, and if sensitive to autonomic or vasoactive substances, take part in an arterial shunt mechanism diverting blood to the radicular arteries. Intra-osseous arterial shunts have been demonstrated in the long bones of rabbits in response to exercise (Pooley et al, 1984) and in dogs and mice after the administration of noradrenalin and ATP (McCarthy et al, 1984).

The arterial supply to the spinal cord, and presumably the cauda equina, are subject to vasodilatation in response to muscle activity. Blau and Rushworth (1958) described local vasodilatation of the ipsilateral regions of the spinal cord of a mouse whose single hind limb was exercised. Similarly, muscular activity in the pre-paralytic stages of poliomyelitis selectively affects the distribution of the paralysis probably from vasodilatation of the anterior horn vessels (Buchthal, 1949). Whether a shunt mechanism assists this vasodilatation is speculative. It would not be unreasonable for the vertebral bodies, which can withstand limited ischaemia, to be temporarily deprived of blood at the expense of the cauda equina during times of intense muscular activity or during hypovolaemic shock.

The lumbar arteries and their branches must be

considered in those cauda equina syndromes which are precipitated by walking. Not infrequently neurogenic and intermittent claudication coexist (Johansson et al, 1982). Atheroma of the abdominal aorta will not only impair flow to the aorto iliac segments, but affect lumbar arterial flow. It will be a factor in the root symptoms if space within the vertebral canal is already at a premium, and there is incipient root ischaemia.

One of the anomalies of the radiculopathies associated with Paget's disease is that the vertebral canal is not invariably narrow (Herzberg and Bayliss, 1980, Ravinchandran, 1981). A vertebral steal syndrome has been suggested as an explanation of the cauda equina symptoms, which is sometimes reversible with calcitonin therapy (Walpin and Singer, 1979, Douglas et al, 1981). The intraosseous branches of the lumbar arteries cannot be neglected when considering cauda equina ischaemia as a pain source.

The complicated venous channels in the extradural compartment of the vertebral canal (Batson's plexus, 1940), freely communicate with the azygos system of veins by the radicular veins. They accompany the nerve roots in the root canal through the intervertebral foramen. The communicating radicular veins are without valves, and thus the pressure within the vertebral canal is increased with raised intra abdominal pressure. A patient who already has back pain from some lesion within the vertebral canal where limitation of space is a problem, is likely to have an increase in that pain when the venous pressure increases. Coughing, straining and lifting, will increase that pressure, and the same mechanism may explain some types of pre-menstrual back pain.

Some patients with neurogenic claudication have significant epidural venous engorgement which can add to the surgical difficulties. Degenerative change in the vertebral bodies with increased interosseous venous pressure may be of some importance in this syndrome. Vertebral veins draining into Batson's plexus will increase the epidural pressure during exercise. The reduction of venous pressure could explain the rapid recovery of impending paraplegia in some patients with Paget's disease when treated with calcitonin (Douglas et al, 1981) and the same drug's effect on some patients with neurogenic claudication (Porter and Hibbert, 1983).

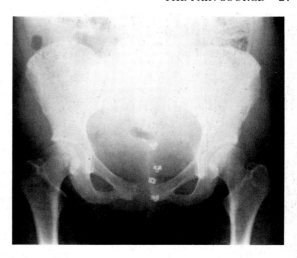

Fig. 4.5 Showing spontaneous disruption of the pubic symphysis after an obstructed labour was relieved by a Caesarean section. The patient complained of back pain and had difficulty walking for a few weeks.

THE SACRO-ILIAC JOINT

The sacro-iliac joint is a large joint of irregular contour, supported by powerful ligaments. It is unusual for it to be a source of pain following a mechanical injury. Sacro-iliac over-use may cause pain in military recruits with a positive scintiscan (Chising et al, 1984) but for most patients who complain of pain in the sacro-iliac region, a careful assessment of the lumbar spine usually confirms that this is referred from the mid line. Serious disruption of the sacro iliac joint can accompany pelvic fractures and separation of the public symphysis. In those countries where obstructed labour is relieved by symphysiotomy and in spontaneous disruption of the symphisis, sacro iliac pain can persist for months (Fig. 4.5). Over-enthusiastic removal of donor bone from the posterior ileum will cause longstanding pain and tenderness if the joint is transgressed, but these instances are rare when considering the total back pain population.

The sacro-iliac joint is often the first joint of the axial skeleton to be affected by inflammatory disorders. It may produce the first symptom of ankylosing spondylitis, and sub-clinical forms with intermittent back pain but no abnormal radiological signs, may be relatively common in both sexes. Pain and tenderness in the sacro-iliac region may follow pelvic infection in women and prostatitis in men, with the appearance of osteitis condensans ilii. The joint is not easily disturbed, however, by mechanical derangement.

There is no consensus of agreement about the source of pain in most back pain syndromes, but it is not improbable that patients with a back pain problem of mechanical origin experience pain from two main sources 1) tissues which restrain shear, or 2) tissues within the vertebral canal, especially the dura, ganglia and roots. This at least supports the known facts and provides a working basis for understanding many back pain mechanisms. We shall look at these in detail.

REFERENCES

Attenborough C G, Reynolds M T 1975 Lumbo-sacral fusion with spring fixation. Journal of Bone and Joint Surgery 57-B: 283–288

Batson O V 1940 The function of the vertebral veins and their role in the spread of metastases. Annals of Surgery 112: 138–149

Blau J N, Rushworth G 1958 Observations of blood vessels of the spinal cord and their response to motor activity. Brain 81: 354–363

Bogduk N, Tynan W, Wilson A S 1981 The nerve supply to the human lumbar intervertebral discs. Journal of Anatomy 132: 39

Buchthal F 1949 Problems of the pathologic physiology of poliomyelitis. American Journal of Medicine 6: 597–591

Caplan L R, Kleeman F J, Berg S 1977 Urinary retention probably secondary to herpes genetalis. New England Journal of Medicine Vol 297: No. 17, 920–921

Chisin R, Milgrom C, Margulies J, Giladi M, Stein M, Kashtan H, Atlan H 1984 Unilateral sacroiliac overuse syndrome in military recruits. British Medical Journal 289: 590–591

Cyriax J 1978 Dural Pain. The Lancet, April 29, 1978, 919–921

Domminisse G F 1975 The arteries and veins of the human spinal canal from birth. Edinburgh Churchill Livingstone

Douglas D L, Duckworth T, Kanis J A, Jefferson A A, Martin T J, Russell R G G 1981 Spinal cord dysfunction in Paget's disease of bone: has medical treatment a vascular basis? Journal of Bone and Joint Surgery 63–B: 495–503

Herzberg L, Bayliss E 1980 Spinal cord syndrome due to non-compressible Paget's disease of bone: a spinal artery steal phenomenon reversible with calcitonin. Lancet 1980, Vol 2: 13–15

Johansson J E, Barrington T W, Ameli M 1982 Combined vascular and neurogenic claudication. Spine 7: 150–158

Kadish L J and Simmons E H 1984 Anomalies of the lumbosacral nerve roots: an anatomical investigation and myelographic study. Journal of Bone and Joint Surgery 66–B: 411–416

Leyshon A, Kirwan E O'G, Wynn Parry C B 1980 Is it nerve root pain? Journal of Bone and Joint Surgery 62–B: 119

McCarthy I D, Davies R, Hughes S P F 1984 The response of the microcirculation in bone to the administration of noradrenaline and ATP. Presented to the British Orthopaedic Research Society, Stanmore 1984.

McCall I W, Park W M, O'Brien J P 1979 Induced pain referred from posterior lumbar elements in normal subjects. Spine 4: 441–446

Pooley J, Pooley J E and Stevens J 1984 Evidence for an intraosseous arteriovenous shunt operating in long bones during exercise conditions. Presented to the British Orthopaedic Research Society Stanmore, 1984

Porter R W, Hibbert C 1983 Calcitonin treatment for neurogenic claudication. Spine 8: 585–592

Ratcliffe J F 1980 The arterial anatomy of the adult human lumbar vertebral body. A microarteriographic study. Journal of Anatomy 131: 57–79

Ratcliffe J F 1981 The arterial anatomy of the developing human dorsal and lumbar vertebral body. A microarteriographic study. Journal of Anatomy 133: 625–638

Ratcliffe J F 1982 An evaluation of the intra-osseous arterial anastomoses in the human vertebral body at different ages. A microarteriographic study. Journal of Anatomy 134: 373–382

Ravichandran G 1981 Spinal cord function in Paget's disease of spine. Paraplegia 19: 7–11

Rydevik R 1982 Pathoanatomy and Pathophysiology of Nerve Root Compression. Presented to the Int. Soc. for the Study of the Lumbar Spine, Toronto

Smyth M J and Wright V 1958 Sciatica and the intervertebral disc. Journal of Bone and Joint Surgery 40–A: 1401

Spencer D L, Irwin G S and Miller J A A 1983 Anatomy and significance of fixation of the lumbo-sacral nerve roots in sciatica. Spine 8: 672–679

Walpin L A, Singer F R 1979 Paget's disease, reversal of severe paraparesis with calcitonin. Spine 4: 213–219

Warren K G, Brown et al 1978 Isolation of latent herpes etc. New England Journal of Medicine May, p 1068

Wyke B D 1980 The neurology of low back pain. Chapter 11 in The Lumbar Spine and Back Pain 2nd Edn. p 265–339. Ed. by M I V Jayson, Pitman Medical, London

Yoshizawa H, O'Brien J P, Smith W T et al 1980 The neuropathology of intervertebral disc removed for low back pain. Journal of Pathology 132: 95

Young M H 1973 Long term consequences of stable fractures of the thoracic and lumbar vertebral bodies. Journal of Bone and Joint Surgery 55–B: 295–300

5

The significance of the vertebral canal — and compromise of its contents

The intervertebral disc has enjoyed an era of popularity since Mixter and Barr described the symptoms of an acute disc lesion in 1934. The relative importance of the vertebral canal in the symptomatology of back pain has only gradually been appreciated. Sarpyener (1945) documented 10 patients where a narrow vertebral canal was responsible for deformity and paralytic problems, and then Verbiest in 1954 described the symptoms of neurogenic claudication resulting from spinal stenosis. The available space in the vertebral canal is now recognised as a significant factor in many back pain syndromes, not only in neurogenic claudication, but also root entrapment syndrome, in the acute and chronic disc lesions, and in some of the problems of instability.

ANATOMY

The term 'vertebral canal' refers to a highly complex anatomical space posterior to the vertebral bodies and discs, within the neural arch, which widens and narrows at each vertebral level in both coronal and sagittal plane. There is not only regional variation at each vertebral level, but also considerable individual variation within a population.

The vertebral canal is arbitrarily divided into the central canal and the root canal. At the pedicular level the central canal is bounded laterally by the two pedicles, anteriorly by the posterior surface of the vertebral body, and posteriorly by the cranial aspect of the laminae and the medial aspect of the superior apophyseal joints. Between each pedicular level the central canal has an artificial boundary. It extends

from one pedicular level to the next, and contains the cauda equina within the dural envelope (Fig. 5.1).

The root canal is that space lateral to the central canal, in the intervertebral region between the pedicular levels. Anteriorly it is bounded by the posterior surface of the vertebral body above, the postero-lateral aspect of the disc, and the posterior

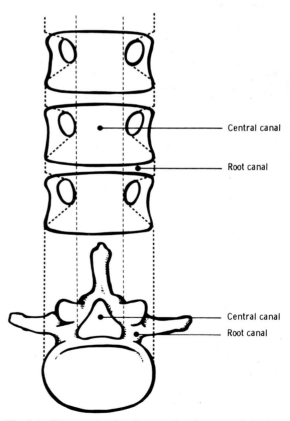

Fig. 5.1 Diagram showing the central and root canals in the coronal and transverse planes.

surface of the vertebral body below. Superiorly it is bounded by the pedicle of the vertebra above, and inferiorly by the pedicle of the vertebra below. Its posterior relations are the lateral aspect of the lamina, and the superior articulation of the apophyseal joint of the vertebra below. Medially it opens into the central canal, and laterally it ends at the intervertebral foramen.

The lateral recess is that lateral part of the central vertebral canal at the pedicular level, anterior to the medial aspect of the superior apophyseal facet (Schatzker and Pennal, 1968). It is only trefoil shaped canals that have a lateral recess, because dome shaped canals have a continuous concave posterior surface to the canal with no lateral recess at all (Fig. 5.2). The root canal has been loosely but inaccurately called the lateral recess.

In the sagittal plane the central canal pursues a serpentine course (Fig. 5.3). It is indented posteriorly by the cranial aspect of each lamina, and anteriorly by each intervertebral disc. In the coronal plane, the vertebral canal is narrowest at each pedicular level, widening into each root canal, and narrowing again at the next pedicular level.

The general dimensions of the vertebral canal tend to follow a constant pattern from the first to the fifth lumbar levels, (Porter et al, 1980). In the mid-sagittal plane at the pedicular level, it is generally widest at L.1, reducing to L.4 and widening again at L.5. In the coronal plane, the inter-pedicular diameter measurements are fairly constant from L.1 to L.3, widening a little at L.4 and then considerably at L.5. The total cross sectional area at the pedicular levels reduces from L.1 to L.4, and then increases at L.5 to an area equal or even greater than at L.1. Measurements from 240 spines are shown in Fig. 5.4. The mean, tenth and ninetieth percentiles are shown for three populations, 119 Romano-British adult spines from Poundbury in the fourth century A.D., 61 spines from Eccles belonging to the sub-Roman and Anglo-Saxon peoples of Kent dating from the mid centuries to the first millenium A.D., and a twentieth century Edinburgh collection of 60 spines mainly of Indian origin. There is considerable variation within each population, with approximately fifty per cent increase in the diameters from the tenth and ninetieth percentiles. The two archaeological collections showed a closer correlation in the anatomy of the vertebral canal. Eisenstein (1977) measuring

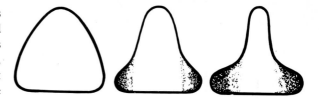

L5 : Central Canal

Fig. 5.2 Diagram to show the variable shape of the central lower lumbar vertebral canal. The dome-shaped canal has no lateral recess, the bell-shaped canal a small recess (shaded), and the trefoil canal a deep lateral recess.

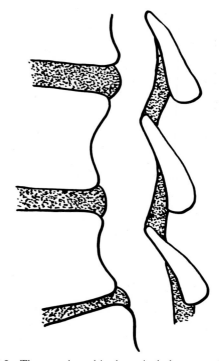

Fig. 5.3 The central canal in the sagittal plane, pursuing a serpentine course.

the mid sagittal diameter of Caucasoid and negro spines found similar absolute measurements with a slight racial difference. The racial variation may have some significance when considering the incidence of back pain syndromes.

The range of mid-sagittal and inter-pedicular diameters is greatest at L.5 with more variability in both size and shape of the canal. Eisenstein (1980) described 14 per cent of canals trefoil at L.5. The trefoil configuration is a relative term caused by postero-lateral indentation of the neural arch. Two extremes of shape at L.5 are shown in Fig. 5.5, but in

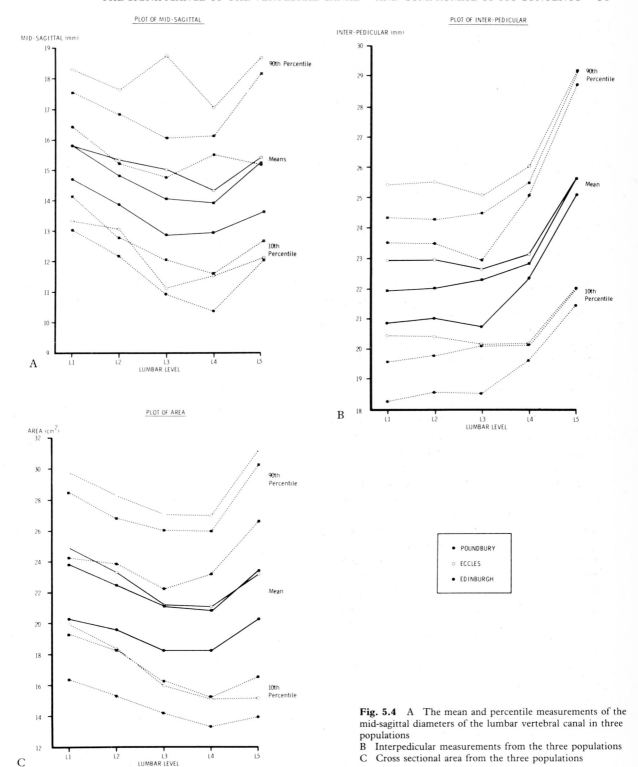

Fig. 5.4 A The mean and percentile measurements of the mid-sagittal diameters of the lumbar vertebral canal in three populations
B Interpedicular measurements from the three populations
C Cross sectional area from the three populations

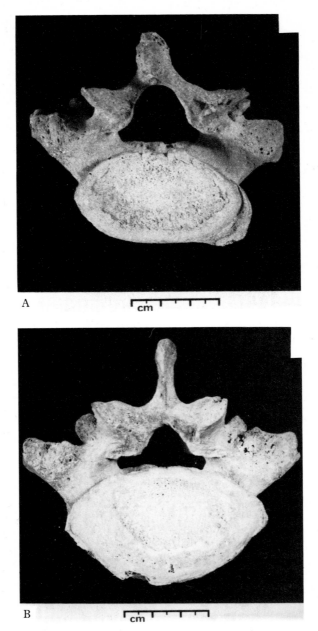

Fig. 5.5 A   Fifth lumbar vertebra viewed from below, showing large bell-shaped vertebral canal.
B   Fifth lumbar vertebra with shallow trefoil shaped vertebral canal..

fact no two canals are the same. We have measured the trefoil configuration of 240 spines using a photographic method (Figs 5.6, 5.7 and 5.8) and it is apparent that the canal of many spines changes to a trefoil shape from L.2 to L.5. The change in shape was fairly constant for the three populations.

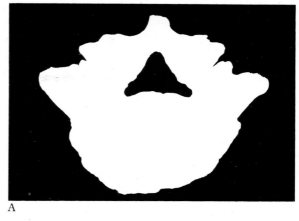

A

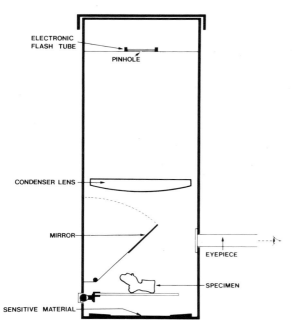

Fig. 5.6 Diagram of a photographic box designed by Mr G Swann, to produce an unmagnified silhouette photograph of the vertebral canal.

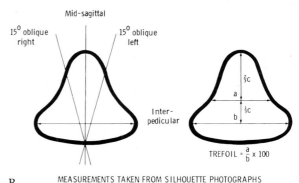

B   MEASUREMENTS TAKEN FROM SILHOUETTE PHOTOGRAPHS

Fig. 5.7 A Silhouette photograph of a fifth lumbar vertebra.
B Measurements taken from silhouette photographs.

One would expect the cross-sectional area of the canal to decrease caudally, as there is a gradual reduction in the volume of the neural contents. At first sight, the increased cross-sectional area at L.5 (Fig. 5.4C) may seem surprising, until we consider the trefoil shape of the canal. A larger cross sectional area will be advantageous when the surface area of the canal increases and in addition, the lordotic curve, most marked at L.5/S.1 places some vulnerability on the neural elements, unless the cross sectional area is increased.

Unfortunately the trefoil shaped canal is unhealthy if that spine is affected by pathological change. Not only are the L.5 nerve roots at risk from encroachment of disc or osteophytes into the lateral recess, but the cross sectional area of trefoil canals is generally less than for non-trefoil canals and the mid sagittal diameter is often reduced (Eisenstein, 1977).

We know little about the cause of the trefoil shaped canal. It is not influenced by the angle of the apophyseal facets, nor by the degree of degenerative change. Baddeley (1976) noted a relationship between the trefoil shape and a vertebra where the pedicle height was small and the apophyseal joints close together. There is, in fact, a correlation of .35 (p < .05) (Table 5.1) but though of interest, this is not sufficient to predict the trefoil shape from a radiograph. There is a better correlation of .50 (p < .05) between the trefoil shape and the degree of wedging of the vertebral body at L.5. It cannot be assumed from a radiograph that a spine with an acute lumbo-sacral angle has a trefoil canal, but it does suggest that lumbar lordosis is a factor in the development of the trefoil shape.

The trefoil shape is uncommon in children under ten years of age, and when it does develop it becomes

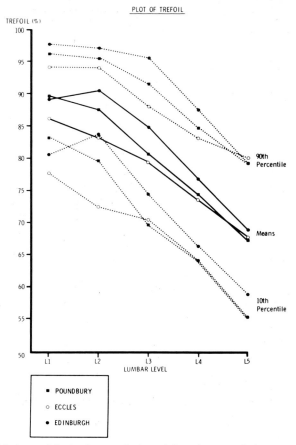

Fig. 5.8   A measure of the trefoil shape of the lumbar vertebral canal from three populations.

Table 5.1   Correlation between the trefoil shape at L.5 and other vertebral measurements.

CORRELATION COEFFICIENT BETWEEN:-

	FACET ANGLE	PEDICLE HEIGHT x FACETAL DISTANCE	WEDGING AT L5	INFERIOR DEGENERATIVE CHANGE	SUPERIOR DEGENERATIVE CHANGE
"TREFOILNESS"	0.04	0.35	0.50	0.30	0.04

apparent in the mid teens. Fig. 5.9 compares the shape of children's and adult's spines and demonstrates a changing shape. If a pliable triangular tube is gradually bent, it will develop a trefoil configuration, which may in fact be the mechanism of some spines becoming trefoil with the development of the secondary curve of lumbar lordosis (Fig. 5.10).

Children's spines

We are surprisingly ignorant about the normal size of the vertebral canal during growth (Haworth and Keillor, 1962, Bowen et al, 1978), but the sagittal diameter does not appear to vary significantly (Larsen and Smith, 1981). Ultrasound measurements of

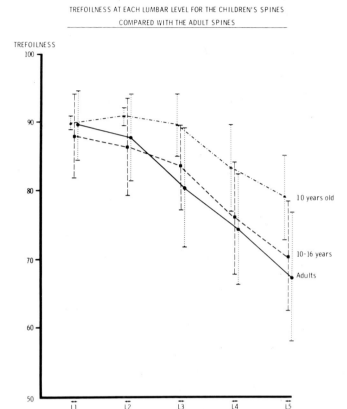

Fig. 5.9 Graph to show the changing trefoil shape of the lumbar vertebral canal with age.

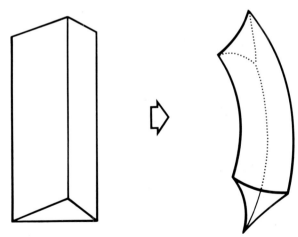

Fig. 5.10 Diagram to show that a triangular tube will develop a trefoil configuration if it is bent.

children's spines suggests that the sagittal diameter is relatively large even in the very young, (Porter et al 1980). The vertebral canal of children appears to be

relatively large when compared with the size of the vertebral body (Fig. 5.11). The size of a child's skull is also relatively large however, and presumably the spinal contents require adequate space. The mid-sagittal and the inter-pedicular diameters of the vertebral canal have approached adult size by the age of ten years, but if the shape is to change, it does so in the years around puberty.

SIGNIFICANCE OF CANAL SIZE

An obvious argument against the vertebral canal being a significant factor in the pathogenesis of back pain, is that although the canal does vary in size and shape from one individual to another, this variation is probably adequate for each subject. In other words, the neural contents may be greater with a large canal, and less with a small canal. The lordotic curve, and the range of movement for one individual may also be

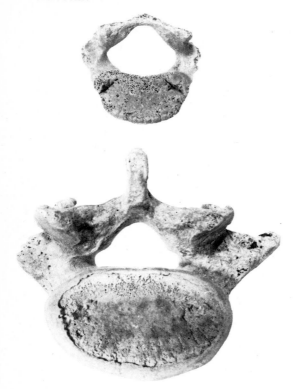

Fig. 5.11 Photograph of a fifth lumbar vertebra of an infant and an adult. A child's canal is relatively large compared with the vertebral body; its cross sectional area approaches that of an adult, but it has different shape.

reflected in the canal's dimension and be satisfactory for that person. The neural contents undoubtedly influence the dimensions of the vertebral canal to some degree (Roth, 1973), much as the brain determines epigenetically the size of the skull in hydrocephalus and microcephalus (Lindborgh, 1972). In the spine, however, this is not the only factor. There must be other influences at work, both genetic and environmental, because clinical observations show great variation in the proportion of intra dural to extra dural space. We know from CT scans and surgical experience that many patients with back pain have a canal with a small mid sagittal diameter, a trefoil shape and a tightly packed cauda equina. In fact, the canal will often determine the pattern of symptoms from any particular pathology.

Sarpyener (1945), Schlesinger and Taveras (1953), Verbiest (1954), Van Gelderen (1958), the Epsteins (1962), Ehni (1969), Salibi (1976) and many others have described how spinal pathology in the presence of a shallow vertebral canal can produce a variety of back pain syndromes. It is the sagittal diameter rather than the interpedicular diameter that is critical, the exception being in achondroplasia, when a narrow interpedicular diameter can cause stenotic sympotms, (Epstein and Malis, 1955, and Nelson 1970). The argument that the canal size is insignificant because it reflects the contents and is adequate for that individual runs contrary to anatomical and clinical observations.

FACTORS INFLUENCING DEVELOPMENT

Anthropometric measurements could give a clue to the canal's variable shape, but our studies have not really shown any useful correlations. We may expect a tall person to have a large vertebral canal, but this is not in fact the case. There is a relationship between the length of the long bones and the size of the bodies and the inter-pedicular diameter of the vertebral canal. A tall individual does have a wide interpedicular diameter. However, there is no correlation between the mid sagittal diameter and any vertebral or other skeletal measurement (Porter 1980).

There is a weak correlation between the AP and lateral diameters of the skull and the mid sagittal diameter of the canal, but this is not sufficient to accurately predict the canal size from skull measurement. Perhaps it reflects a weak epigenetic influence of the neural contents on the canal's size.

The clinically important mid-sagittal diameter of the vertebral canal is independent of other anthropmetric measurements — it cannot be predicted, and must be measured directly.

We found a useful multiple correlation coefficient of .67 (p < .01) with the trefoil canal at L5 and a large calf inequality, inequality of calf to heel measurement and a small biacromial diameter (Porter, 1980). Twin studies suggest that these parameters are affected by environment, and therefore the trefoil canal may also be the result of adverse environment.

There is an inter-relationship between the morphology of the vertebral canal at different levels. Measurements from over 1600 specimens showed that the cross sectional area of the lumbar vertebral canal correlates fairly well with that of the cervical spine (r = .65 p < 0.001), at least for the upper and mid lumbar levels (Table 5.2), and the interpedicular

Table 5.2 Table showing correlations between cross sectional area of lumbar and cervical vertebral canals, with significance of p<.001 marked (X). The best correlations were between L.1 and C.3 and L.2 and C.2.

Area

	C2	C3	C4	C5	C6	C7
L1	✗	✗ r = .65	✗	✗	✗	✗
L2	✗ r = .64	✗	✗	✗	✗	✗
L3		✗	✗	✗		✗
L4	✗	✗	✗	✗		✗
L5						✗

Table 5.4 Table showing correlations between mid-sagittal diameters of lumbar and cervical vertebral canals, the best being between C.7 and L.5 and C.3 and C.7.

Mid-Sagittal Diameter

	C2	C3	C4	C5	C6	C7
L1						
L2	✗					✗
L3	✗	✗	✗		✗	✗
L4	✗		✗		✗	
L5	✗	✗ r = .54	✗	✗	✗	✗ r = .31

diameters at the mid cervical and mid lumbar levels also show a useful correlation (Table 5.3). It is interesting that the mid sagittal diameters correlate only between the cervical and lower lumbar levels (r = 0.54 between C.3 and L.5, p<0.001), (Table 5.4), levels of both cervical and lumbar regions which are likely to develop pathological change (Porter et al, 1983, Rothman, 1972). We need to know much more about the growth and morphology of the vertebral canal, and the factors that influence it.

Clark et al (1984) have suggested that because the vertebral canal completes 90 per cent of its growth by late infancy, factors which disrupt growth before late infancy may have a pronounced and irreversible effect on the adult canal size. They recorded smaller canals in a Mississipian population of skeletons, which had suffered from infant malnutrition, when compared with a hunting and gathering pre-Mississipian population. Our measurements from Indian skeletons

Table 5.3 Table showing correlations between interpedicular diameters of lumbar and cervical vertebral canals, the best being between L.3 and L.4 with C.3 and C.4.

Inter-pedicular Diameter

	C1	C2	C3	C4	C5	C6	C7
L1		✗	✗	✗	✗	✗	✗
L2	✗	✗	✗	✗	✗	✗	✗
L3	✗	✗	✗ r = .42	✗ r = .43	✗	✗	✗
L4		✗	✗ r = .41	✗ r = .43	✗	✗	
L5					✗		✗

would tend to support this concept, though it is difficult to establish nutritional standards from archaeological studies.

Malcomb (1981) has suggested that because body tissues are crystalline in structure, it is to be expected that their growth would resemble that of crystals and liquid crystals. Crystal spirals are logarithmic, as in the spiral growth commonly found in sea shells, and the shape of the human ribs fits well into a hexagonal logarithmic spiral. Spirals may occur of opposite sense and when conjoined produce a variety of forms, and re-entrant angles be a source of self perpetuating growth steps. He suggests that the complicated shape of the vertebrae may be explained in terms of crystal growth. It may yet account for variations in form.

PATHOLOGICAL CHANGE

There is no evidence that the mid-sagittal or the inter-pedicular diameters of the vertebral canal reduce with age after puberty. However, degenerative change at the margins of the apophyseal joints can encroach into the vertebral canal, especially the root canal, and osteophytes can develop from the cranial edge of the laminae into the ligamentum flavum, Fig. 5.12. A posterior vertebral bar can develop at the cranial or caudal aspect of the posterior surface of the vertebral bodies, generally in association with disc degeneration, but the central bony canal is probably not reduced in diameter by age related processes. Skeletal studies have not shown any reduction in canal

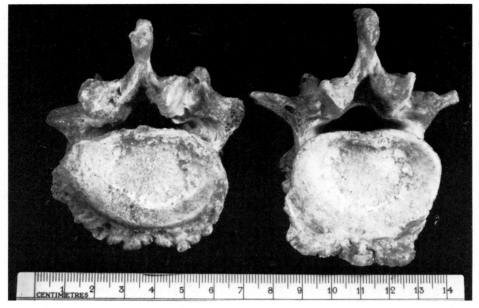

Fig. 5.12 A fifth lumbar vertebra on the left, showing degenerative change of the apophyseal joints encroaching into the root canal, osteophytes at the attachment of the ligamentum flavum, and a posterior vertebral bar of bone. The right hand specimen shows the adjacent fourth lumbar vertebra with a shallow trefoil central canal, not affected by the degenerative change.

diameters in older spines, nor have in vivo studies of different occupational groups.

Soft tissue changes can certainly reduce the capacity of the vertebral canal. CT imaging has shown that the ligamentum flavum may become thickened and buckle into the posterior margin of the central canal and root canal. The anterior margin of the canal may be indented by the posterior longitudinal ligamentum overlying bulging degenerate discs or by previously sequestrated disc material, and iatrogenic scarring can also reduce the canal's capacity.

The canal is also deformed by segmental movement, or vertebral displacement in any of the three planes of rotation.

Thus, although the bony canal does not become narrower with age, age related processes, degeneration and injury can significantly compromise an already narrow canal.

The vertebral canal is one factor that cannot be ignored when attempting to understand the mechanism of a patient's back pain. What is its size and shape? Could there be clinically significant disproportion between the contents and the capacity of the central or the root canal? How important are the soft tissues, vertebral displacement or unnatural segmental movement? It is only as these questions are answered that the diagnosis of a patient's back pain, and eventually its management, become possible. Think space.

REFERENCES

Baddeley H 1976 Radiology of lumbar spinal stenosis. The Lumbar Spine and Back Pain, Pitman Medical Publishing Company 151–171

Bowen V, Shannan R, Kirkcaldy-Willis W H 1978 Lumbar spinal stenosis. Child's Brain 4: 257–277

Clark G A, Panjabi M M and Wetzel F T 1984 Infant malnutrition and adult spinal stenosis. Presented to the International Society for Study of the Lumbar Spine Montreal.

Ehni G 1969 Significance of the small lumbar spinal canal: cauda equina compression syndrome due to spondylolysis. Journal of Neurology 31: 490–494

Eisenstein S 1977 Morphometry and pathological anatomy of the lumbar spine in South African negroes and caucasoids with specific reference to spinal stenosis. Journal of Bone and Joint Surgery, 59–B: 173–180

Eisenstein S 1980 The trefoil configuration of the lumbar vertebral canal. Journal of Bone and Joint Surgery 62–B: 73–77

Epstein J A, Malis L I 1955 Compression of spinal cord and cauda equina in achondroplastic dwarfs. Neurology 5: 875–881

Epstein J A, Epstein B S, Levine I 1962 Nerve root compression associated with narrowing of the lumbar spinal canal. Journal of Neurology, Neurosurgery and Psychiatry 25: 165–176

Haworth J B, Keillor G W 1962 Use of transparencies in evaluating the width of the spinal canal in infants, children and adults. Radiology 79, 109–114

Larsen J L, Smith D 1981 The lumbar spinal canal in children. European Journal of Radiology 1: 163–170

Lindborgh J V 1972 The role of genetic and local environmental factors in the control of post natal craniofacial morphogenesis. Acta Morphologica Neth-Scandonavica 10: 37–47

Malcomb J E 1981 Crystalline structure of the vertebral column: thoracic region. Journal of Anatomy 133: 148–150

Mixter W J, Barr J S 1934 Rupture of the intervertebral disc with involvement of the spinal canal. The New England Journal of Medicine 211: 210–215

Nelson M A, 1970 Orthopaedic aspects of the chondrodystrophies. Annals of the Royal College of Surgeons of England 47: 185–210

Porter R W 1980. Measurement of the lumbar spinal canal by diagnostic ultrasound. MD Thesis. University of Edinburgh

Porter R W, Hibbert C, Wellman P 1980 Backache and the lumbar spinal canal. Spine: Vol 2, No.8 March/April 1980

Porter R W, Hibbert C, Evans C 1983 Relationship between the cervical and lumbar spinal canal. Annals of the Royal College of Surgeons of England, 65: 334

Roth M 1973 The relative osteo-neural growth. A concept of normal and pathological (tetrogenic) skeletal morphogenesis. Gegenbaurs morph. Jahrb., Leipzig 119: 250–274

Rothman H R 1972 The patho-physiology of disc degeneration. Clinical neurosurgery. Proceedings at the Congress of Neurological Surgeons 1972

Salibi B S 1976 Neurogneic claudication and stenosis of the lumbar spinal canal. Surgical Neurology 5: 269–272

Sarpyener M A 1945 Congenital stricture of the spinal canal. Journal of Bone and Joint Surgery 27: 70–79

Schatzker J, Pennal G F 1968 Spinal stenosis, a cause of cauda equina compression. The Journal of Bone and Joint Surgery 50–B: 606–618

Schlesinger E B, Taveras J M 1953 Factors in the production of cauda equina syndromes in lumbar discs. Transactions of the American Neurological Association 78: 263

Van Gelderen V 1958 Ein Orthotisches (lordotisches) kauda syndrom. Acta Psychiatr. Neurol Scand 23: 57

Verbiest H 1954 A radicular syndrome from developmental narrowing of the lumbar vertebral canal. Journal of Bone and Joint Surgery 36–B: 230

6

Structures that restrain shear — and their failure

A second major source of back pain is the failure of structures that restrain shear. The spine moves as one intact unit, flexing extending and rotating as a flexible rod. Forward displacement can occur if the shear forces are not adequately restrained. In the upright posture the disc space between L.3 and L.4 is horizontal (Farfan, 1973), but the intervertebral segment L.4/5 and especially L.5/S.1 are subject to shearing forces (Fig. 6.1). These forces are restrained by the apophyseal joint, by the intact disc, by paraspinal muscles and ligaments and by the abdominal

pressure. This is adequate to prevent segmental displacement in normal conditions.

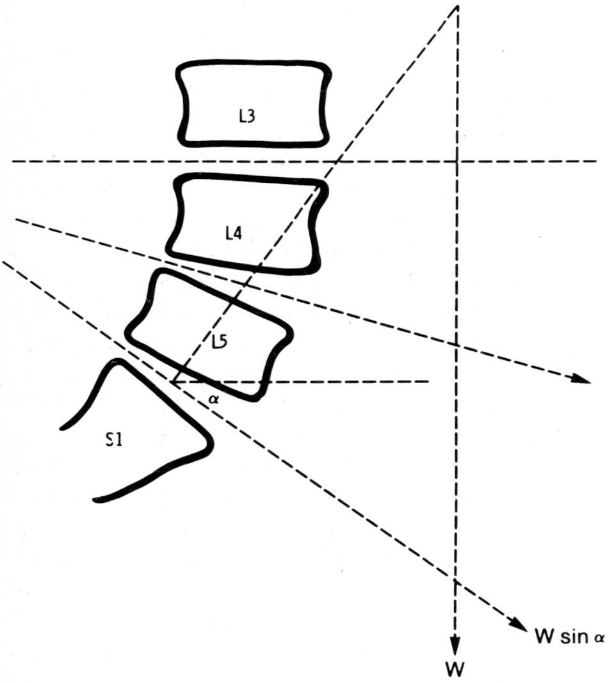

THE APOPHYSEAL JOINTS RESTRAIN SHEAR

They are orientated towards the sagittal plane in the upper lumbar spine, and more coronally at the lower lumbar levels. The mean measurements for 119 skeletons is shown in Table 6.1. The angle of inclination is difficult to measure, because the joints are curved in the two planes and in the transverse plane they tend to form the arc of a circle. In the upper lumbar spine, the sagittal orientation restrains rotation, but permits flexion and extension. The apophyseal joints do not need to restrain forward shear in the upper lumbar spine, except in positions of flexion. The coronal orientation of the joints in the lower lumbar spine is a powerful restraint to shear (Farfan, 1978) and at L.5 the torque is buttressed by

Fig. 6.1 Diagram to show shear through the lumbo-sacral disc, where W is the body weight above and disc, and α the lumbosacral angle.

Table 6.1 Mean measurement of the superior lumbar facet angle of 119 skeletons.

	Mean Facet Angle (degrees)	
LI	66.5	± 13.3
L2	61.3	6.8
L3	54.4	10.0
L4	41.5	10.8
L5	38.8	7.4

the broad pedicles of L.5. The inclination of these lower joints does not prevent rotation as effectively as at upper lumbar levels. The restraint to shear is at the expense of rotation, significant perhaps in disc pathology.

It has been suggested that asymmetrical orientation of the apophyseal joints may be a prelude to disc degeneration (Farfan et al, 1973, and Cyron and Hutton 1980). 28 per cent of our series had asymmetry between the L.5 facets of more than five degrees (Table 6.2). Asymmetry may be the initiating factor in some patients developing rotational instability.

Table 6.2 Percentage of vertebrae with facet asymmetry greater than 5 degrees, and the mean difference between these facet angles.

	More than 5 degrees asymmetrical facets	Mean Difference for these facets (degrees)
LI	21%	10. 4
L2	26%	9. 0
L3	34%	10. 4
L4	32%	9. 8
L5	28%	10. 1

We correlated facet tropism with asymmetry of the vertebral canal, and with rotation of the canal in respect to the vertebral body, but found no useful correlation in 119 skeletons. Nor did degenerative change measured by the size of the vertebral body osteophytes correlate with either the degree of asymmetry of the facet joints or with the angle of the joint at that level. If asymmetry does predispose an individual to rotational displacement, then it is either not necessarily associated with degenerative change, or it is so infrequent an occurrence that it was not detected in this series of specimens.

The most frequent site for degenerative spondylolisthesis is at L.4/5 where the shearing forces are not adequately restrained by the apophyseal joints. Microfractures and remodelling occurs in the subchondral bone of the joints. The vertebra slowly displaces forwards, with gradual bony deformity, loss of disc integrity and stretching of the ligaments. The causative factors and their related importance are uncertain. Possibly osteoporosis is significant, the sagittal orientation of the joints and disruption of the disc. There is no evidence that joint laxity is significant.

An intact neural arch is essential for the apophyseal joints to effectively restrain shear. The fact that spondylolysis can be present with no vertebral displacement, suggests that spinal structures other than the neural arch play a significant part in resisting shear forces.

DISC INTEGRITY RESTRAINS SHEAR

An intact disc restrains shear. Many discs fail and become degenerate without the occurrence of vertebral displacement. It is probable, however, that an intact disc, with adjacent anterior and posterior longitudinal ligaments, supplements other structures in resisting shear (Troup, 1975).

MUSCULO-LIGAMENTOUS COMPLEX RESTRAINS SHEAR

The apophyseal joint capsules, the anterior and posterior longitudinal ligaments, the supra spinous, interspinous and inter transverse ligaments, the lumbar fascia with muscle attachments, the strong lumbo sacral ligament between the fifth lumbar transverse process and the sacrum are in combination efficient restrainers of shear. The para-spinal muscles within the envelopes of the three layers of the lumbar fascia and the psoas muscle anteriorly provide a splint to support the spine, reinforced by intra-abdominal pressure. It is probable that this musculo-ligamentous complex prevents further forward displacement occurring in lytic spondylolisthesis, after cessation of growth. In spite of bilateral pars defects at L.5, there is little further displacement even though the forces of shear remain. It probably is prevented by the soft tissue restraint, especially the lumbo-sacral ligament, and an intact disc.

Ligamentous laxity that accompanies pregnancy in the last trimester (Calgurneri et al, 1982) increases the risk of injury from the increasing shear forces. Not a few women date their first onset of back pain to pregnancy.

The failure to adequately restrain shear may affect many of the pain sensitive tissues of the spine, especially with fatigue pain of the musculo-tendinous complex, and subluxation pain of the apophyseal joints. These are discussed in Chapter 15; it is a second major source of back pain.

REFERENCES

Calguneri M, Bird H A and Wright V 1982 Changes in joint laxity occurring during pregnancy. Annals of the Rheumatic Diseases 41: 126–128

Cyron R M, Hutton W C 1980 Articular trophism and stability of the lumbar spine. Spine 5: 168–172

Farfan H F 1973 The mechanical disorders of the lower back. Philadelphia, Lea and Febiger

Farfan H F 1978 The biochemical advantage of lordosis and hip extension for upright man as compared with other anthropoids. Spine 3: 336

Troup J D G 1975 Mechanical factors in spondylolisthesis and spondylolysis. Clinical Orthopaedics and Related Research 117: 59–67

7

Pain perception and pain behaviour

A sensory stimulus above a certain threshold can become a pain source, but that pain stimulus is considerably modified by the nocioceptive system, before it becomes perceived as pain. The same pain source will produce different pain perception in different subjects and in the same subject at different times. This is apparent in many situations. Two patients having identical operations will estimate their pain perception very differently, and have variable post-operative analgesic requirements. In fact, the same patient having sequential bilateral procedures will frequently comment that for some unexplained reason one operation was more painful than the other. Two individuals with apparently identical fractures will assess their pain very differently, some experiencing little discomfort, and others feeling intense pain, with no obvious explanation from the pain source. The nervous system between the receptor and the higher centres has considerable potential to modify pain in the so-called 'nocioceptive system' so that pain perception is not directly proportional to the stimulus.

THE POSTERIOR HORN

The posterior horn cell does not simply receive a sensory stimulus from the peripheral afferent fibre and pass it to higher centres in an unmodified form. In the posterior horn of the spinal cord there are probably side circuits which can excite or prolong the activity of the original impulse with secondary circuits able to inhibit the transmission of the impulse. Substance 'P', neurotensin, oxytocin, encephalins and other peptides have been identified in many of the intermediary cells of the posterior horn of the spinal cord, substances which have an ability to modify the impulses received by sensory afferents from the pain source.

This concept explains the reduction in pain perception by such activities as rubbing the skin over a painful site, by applying local heat to a painful area, and it explains the benefits of massage, the application of vibrators, and transcutaneous nerve stimulation. These all stimulate mechano-receptors which could produce an inhibitory effect on pain at the posterior horn level. These observations in practice are supported by neuro-physiological studies (Wall, 1979) and although the pathways have not been identified, and they have not received universal acceptance (Schmidt, 1972), it would seem that their presence is most probable. The activity of the nocioceptive complex in the posterior horn is probably modified by a control mechanism from higher centres. Thus a stimulus can be conducted from the pain source by the peripheral nerve to the posterior horn synapse, but because of modification at the posterior horn level, on one occasion the pain perception may be intense from summation or prolongation, and on another occasion, the same stimulus may result in minimal pain perception from a variety of inhibitory mechanisms.

The substantia gelatinosa is the most likely site of the spinal gating mechanism (Melzack and Wall, 1965). It receives axon terminals from many of the large and small diameter fibres and the dendrites of the cells in the deeper laminae project into it. It also forms a functional unit that extends the length of the spinal cord on each side, its cells interconnecting by short fibres influencing distal sites. This anatomical arrangement may explain an interesting phenomenon when patients with pain in one lower limb experience sensory disturbance in the ipsilateral but rarely in the contralateral upper limb. The spinal gating mechanism may modulate conduction of nerve impulses over many segments.

THE MID BRAIN

Modification of pain was first recognised by animal experimentation, when stimulation of the peri-aqueductal grey matter made the animal unresponsive to pain. Subsequently it was observed that the injection of radioactive labeled morphine was identified at precisely the same area of the mid brain. The identification of enkephalin, and other morphine-like substances the endorphines, manufactured in the peri-aqueductal grey matter and released by electrical stimulation at this site, suggests a mid-brain system of pain inhibition (Kosierlitz et al, 1977, Terenius and Wahlstrom, 1979). Nalorphine blocks the effects of morphine by being so similar to the morphine molecule that it can become attached in the mid brain to the specific morphine receptor. The peripheral pain stimulus is then consciously perceived. There exists a complex mid-brain system of pain modification before pain is experienced as an abnormal unpleasant sensation.

The control of this mid-brain system of pain modification has yet to be resolved, but it does explain the apparent absence of pain experienced by casualties in war, by boxers, by athletes enduring ischaemic pain, and a large percentage of the population arriving at the dentist's surgery. Certainly they have a pain source, but a modified pain perception, at least temporarily.

Pain enhancement

We are aware therefore of the possibility of a pain stimulus with no pain perception, and can perhaps explain its mechanism. When dealing with some patients suffering from severe back pain, we ask whether it is possible to have pain perception with no continuing pain source. Experiments under hypnosis would suggest that it is, when pain can be genuinely experienced from an imaginary source. Thirty-five per cent of amputees suffer from phantom pain (Feinsein et al, 1954) though the stump is usually healthy and there is no obvious pain source. Melzack and Wall (1965) explained spontaneous pain of causalgia and neuralgia in terms of a summation

mechanism. The pain experience is not a 'one to one' relationship with the stimulus.

CONSCIOUS PAIN

When pain is perceived at conscious level, it has three recognisable components, described by the Hilgards (1975) as sensory pain, suffering and mental anguish. Sensory pain is simply the appreciation of a sensory stimulus as pain. The suffering component involves the frontal cortex. When fibres from the thalamus to the frontal cortex are transected by orbito-frontal leucotomy, the subject is still aware of the sensory stimulus of pain, but the suffering element is largely removed. He is no longer 'in pain' (Freeman and Watts, 1950, Mark et al, 1963). The 'mental anguish' component of pain is associated with anxiety and a complexity of emotions, with a resultant pattern of pain behaviour (Gibson, 1982). It is this objective response of the patient to the original pain source, their pain behaviour, that the clinician observes. This psychological component is uniquely individual. That is, the same pain experience can be expected to produce a very different individual behavioural response.

An individual's response to pain will depend on inherited characteristics, previous environmental experience, and the present situation, not least the meaning ascribed to the sensation, and an intellectual assessment of the probable outcome of different response strategies. The psychological traits of phobia, anxiety, depression, obsession, hysteria, or a tendency to somatise will be influenced by genetic characteristics, and the imprinting of life's early experiences in infancy and childhood. A child who finds illness rewarding by receiving parental attention, and being able to escape the demands of school, may look for benefits from pain in later life. A more disciplined childhood, with demands for a 'stiff upper lip' can produce a stoical attitude to pain. Certainly ethnic groups have contrasting behavioural responses to back pain, when the anatomical and pathological variations seem relatively insignificant (Bremner et al, 1968, Eisenstein, 1977, and Glass, 1979). Many fears and anxieties in adult life are projections from childhood. The observation of a child on his parents attitude to pain will influence his behaviour. The sins of the father are visited on his children to the third and fourth generation.

The immediate environmental situation also will influence the behaviour to pain, the response of the spouse, family, friends and colleagues at work. Behaviour will be affected by the rewards of attention or lack of it from doctors and therapists, by financial benefits and the opportunity to avoid unpleasant work. It is not affected by social class (Larson and Marcer, 1984).

It is as important to ask: 'What kind of patient has back pain' as 'What kind of back pain has this patient'. The influence of many known and unknown factors on the patient's basic psychological character will produce a variable response. The obsessional individual may have little time to dwell on pain, and neglect the conscious pain experience. If on the other hand an anxiety state is superimposed on the obsessional character, the pain may become exaggerated and new symptoms added. Depression or phobia may cause abnormal pain behaviour, or prolong its course.

A readiness to somatise in adverse circumstances may cause a patient to seek medical help for pain which others would manage alone, (Wolkind and Forrest, 1972). We carried out an epidemiological study of the incidence of attendances for back pain in four general practices, examining the records of over four hundred men and their wives over 40 years of age and covering an average period of 20 years. The mean attendance rate for conditions other than back pain, was significantly higher for both men and women who attended with back pain, than for those individuals who never attended with back pain (Table 7.1). Becker and Karch (1979) similarly observed that patients complaining of low back pain are a group who present their symptoms to doctors more readily than other individuals.

We noted in this series that the role of the spouse is highly important in pain behaviour. Husbands and wives tended to polarise, those men and women who were high attenders with back pain, having a spouse who was a low attender (Table 7.2).

Table 7.2 Comparative mean general practice attendance rate per year for all conditions, for wives of 40 year old miners who had above average attendance rate for all conditions, and wives of miners with below average attendance rate, over a 20 year period (n = 96)

	Wives attendance rate per year for all conditions
Miners whose attendance rate for all conditions per year was above average (6.01 visits/year).	2.97
Miners whose attendance rate for all conditions per year was below average (2.53 visits/year)	4.08

ASSESSMENT OF PAIN BEHAVIOUR

A clinician treating patients with back pain eventually develops an intuitive sense about pain behaviour. From the manner in which the patient enters the consulting room, the way he walks, sits, talks, his facial expression, they all give a hint of appropriate or inappropriate behaviour, which is then supported by the examination (Waddell, 1979, and Leavitt et al, 1979). Most patients fall into the middle ground of what would be considered an acceptable response to pain. A few have an exaggerated response, more so if the history is long. These we can identify but we are less skilled at recognising the stoic.

We can identify the exaggerating patient who has a small or non-existent organic pain source (page 54). That does not mean that there was not originally some mechanical failure of the spine, a genuine source of pain and a pain experience. With the passage of time the organic cause can cease, but the experience remains. We are not dealing with malingering. Symptoms persist when they seem to have no gainful value, when litigation has been settled.

Recognising inappropriate behaviour warns the clinician that he is faced not only with a complex diagnostic problem, but difficult management. Sophisticated investigations may be counter-productive, and some methods of treatment positively harmful. We recognise a problem but can rarely modify and change it.

Table 7.1 Comparison between mean attendances for conditions other than back pain for 403 men with and without back pain

	Men with Back Pain. (n = 255) Mean attendance per year for conditions other than Back Pain	Men without Back Pain. (n = 148) Mean attendance per year with other conditions
Mining Practice A	5.57 (SD 3.98)	3.22 (SD 2.47)
Mining Practice B	6.01 (SD 7.67)	3.65 (SD 2.71)
Town Practice A	3.34 (SD 2.45)	2.22 (SD 1.87)
Town Practice B	2.57 (SD 1.85)	1.74 (SD 2.08)

Attempting to identify the source of back pain, by observing a patient's pain behaviour, can in no way be compared to identifying a fault in a machine. Modification at spinal mid-brain and cortical level is to such a degree that it is a wonder that a pain source can be discovered at all. Fortunately, in spite of the fascinating complexity of the nocioceptive system, and the factors that influence the patient's behaviour, the majority of patients respond to their pain in a rational appropriate manner. What they experience is in proportion to the organic lesion, and their behaviour is not exaggerated. It is upon this premise that we attempt to make a reasonable diagnosis of the cause of the pain.

REFERENCES

Becker L A, Karch F 1979 Low back pain in family practice: a case control study. The Journal of Family Practice 9: 579–582

Bremner J M, Lawrence J S, Miall W E 1968 Degenerative joint disease in a Jamaican rural population. Annals of the Rheumatic Diseases 27: 327–332

Eisenstein S 1977 Morphometry and pathological anatomy of the lumbar spine in South African negroes and caucasoids with specific reference to spinal stenosis. Journal of Bone and Joint Surgery, 59-B: 173–180

Feinstain B, Luce J C, Langton J N K 1954 The influence of phantom limbs in P Wilson and P Klopsteg (eds). Human limbs and their substitutes McGraw-Hill

Freeman W and Watts J W 1950 Psychosurgery in the treatment of mental disorders and intractable pain. Thomas, Springfield, Ill

Gibson H B 1982 Pain and its conquest. Peter Owen, London and Boston

Glass J B 1979 Acute lumbar strain. Clinical signs and prognosis. The Practitioner 222: 821–825

Hilgard E R and Hilgard J R 1975 Hypnosis in the relief of pain. Los Altos, Calif. W. Kaufmann p.29

Kosierlitz H W, Hughes J, Law J H, Waterfield J A 1977 Encephalins, endorphines and opiate receptors. Nerosci Symp Vol 2 Society for Neuroscience 291–307

Larson A G, Marcer D 1984 The who and why of pain: analysis by social class. British Medical Journal 288: 883–886

Leavitt F, Garron D C, D'Angelo C M, McNeill T W 1979 Low back pain in patients with or without demonstrable organic disease. Pain 6: 191–200

Mark V H, Ervin F R and Yakolev P I 1963 Stereotactic Thalamotomy. Archives of Neurology 8: 528–538

Melzack R, Wall P D 1965 Pain mechanisms: a new theory. Science 150: 331

Schmidt R F 1972 The gate control theory of pain; an unlikely hypothesis. Payne J P, and Burt R A P, Pain, London, Churchill Livingstone.

Terenius L, Wahlstrom A 1979 Endorphines and clinical pain. An overview. Adv. Exp. Med. Biol. 116: 261–277

Waddell G, McCulloch J A, Kummell E, and Venner R M 1980. Non-organic physical signs in low back pain. Spine 5: 117–125

Wall P D 1979 Modulations of pain by non-painful events. Bonica J J and Albe-Fessard D (eds). Advances in Pain Research and Therapy. New York: Raven Press

Wolkind S N, Forrest A J 1972 Low back pain: a psychosomatic investigation. Postgradulate Medical Journal 48: 76–79

8

The consultation

The clinician's heart should be gladdened, not saddened, by the patient with backache. We have a symptom with so many possible causes in the soma and psyche, that it should challenge our detective skills. Besides the thrill of the chase, we have a condition that will probably get better in spite of us.

There is a danger of becoming too academic, too absorbed by the problem, that we neglect the patient. If he feels like a 'case', an 'interesting condition', a 'statistic in our research programme', we have neglected our primary purpose. We should remind ourselves why the patient seeks a consultation. It is to satisfy the patient, not the doctor. Unless the patient leaves us with a sense of fulfillment, we have failed. McGee (1961) found that 65 per cent of hospital patients were dis-satisfied with the amount of information they received. They want an answer to two questions; What is wrong? and Can you put it right? The whole consultation should encompass these two questions.

But academic we must be. We need to listen, observe, record and learn from this patient's experience in order to unravel the mysteries of back pain. We cannot escape trying to satisfy the doctor because back pain becomes such a fascinating study. From our understanding of this patient, we can help a patient yet to come. The consultation is more than helping the patient before us, important as that is. Back pain has qualities that are probably unique in medicine. Here is a quest to find the elusive cause of a problem, and influence it. We may not be too confident about treating the patient before us, but with every piece of information, every correct observation recorded, assimilated and correctly interpreted, we should gradually improve our understanding and management. Patient care and research are not only mutually compatible, they are complimentary.

The consultation begins as the patient enters the room. It is good psychology to rise and invite the patient to sit down, to sit within a few feet of us, not on the other side of the desk. A smooth flow of conversation is possible if a secretary can unobtrusively record an accurate history without the need to stop for dictation. Give the patient plenty of time (Wright et al, 1982).

1. THE HISTORY

Past history

Generally the patient wants to begin with the recent history, but it helps to direct them to the first episode of back pain perhaps many years before. Not only is this important in appreciating the present problem, but the patient is often pleasantly surprised that someone is at last prepared to listen to the whole story. At what age did they first experience back pain? Did there appear to be a causative episode? We need to know if there was an injury, what was the mechanism, was litigation involved, and what were the subsequent symptoms. We want to know the distribution of pain at that time, if the symptoms affected the back only or the leg, what treatment was offered, and how long it took to recover.

In this history there is generally a clue to the pathology responsible for the first episode of back pain which is relevant to the present problem.

Mrs J.B. first experienced back pain at twenty years of age whilst cleaning at home. She lifted some furniture and twisted, had pain in the back that put her to bed for a week, and she remembers the pain went down to the left foot. It may have been a disc lesion.

Mr J.F. has a lytic spondylolisthesis. He fell off a six feet wall when sixteen years of age. He bruised his lower back and recollects having several months of backache. This is compatible with a disruption of the pars inter-articularis in a pre-existing spondylolisthesis.

Mrs W.H. developed back pain insidiously during the latter part of her second pregnancy, and it was aggravated by her third. The ligamentous laxity of pregnancy and the forces of shear may have caused a segmental mechanical disturbance, which is now a major problem.

Mr H.J. has not worked for four years since he hurt his back at work falling onto the corner of a metal cupboard. The pain affected his back and both legs to the feet. He did not take to his bed but rested at home. The mechanism of the injury, the circumstances surrounding it, and the distribution of pain, would make one consider a non-organic element to the present pain.

Miss K.B., now in her fifties, had no previous history of back pain until three months ago she developed severe pain down to the outer foot. She may have had a previously symptomless disc pathology, and now degenerative change is affecting the root canal.

Although one should be cautious about drawing premature conclusions from the history of the first episode of back pain, it can be invaluable in trying to interpret the present symptoms. They are often the end result of the natural history of a longstanding pathological process.

Intermediate history

The subsequent pattern of pain between the first episode and the present symptoms may help in the prognosis. Has the pattern of pain been getting steadily worse, or is it much the same year after year? We need a clear understanding of its frequency and severity over the years, because there is a fair chance that apart from a change in lifestyle, the coming years will be much the same as the past.

Mr H.K. has been steadily getting more trouble with his back. He left the building trade five years ago, because of a poor work record, and now is aware of fairly constant, increasing backache, in spite of a sedentary job in the office. He is much the same from one day to the next. It is reasonable guess that unless surgery has anything to offer him, the back pain will continue and he will have to give up work altogether.

Over the past six years, Mrs J.B. has had to go to bed two or three times a year with pain in the back and often pain down the right leg to the calf. It generally settles but she has to take care between these attacks. The present episode is no worse than the others. If she cannot modify her life, she will probably carry on with the same periodic pain in the coming years.

Mr L.N. had one episode of back and leg pain five years ago, and has been quite free of pain until last month. His present bout of pain is settling. He could well make a good recovery and have a long spell of freedom.

The factors that influenced pain up to the present episode will also give us some help in future management. Has the patient had pain from obvious abuse of the spine, or in spite of taking reasonable care? The answers to these questions will help us to offer the right advice for the coming years.

Present history

The present episode of back pain, being fresh in the memory, will be described in great detail. The important facts are, how and when did it occur, what has been the distribution of pain, has the distribution changed with time, what factors aggravate the pain, how is it relieved, and is it getting better or worse. At the heart of the history is the daily pattern of pain. It is worth taking the patient through an average day, and if the pain has a mechanical cause, a typical pattern of pain will emerge. If the pain originates from other systems, the gastro-intestinal or gynaecological, it will be related to their particular rhythms. Questions concern the patient's response to getting out of bed, dressing, standing, stooping, sitting, rising from the sitting and stooped position, walking, driving, lifting, carrying, coughing, shopping, activities at home and at work, and the effects of sport. If the cause is mechanical, a typical pattern of pain will emerge from the day's activities to suggest the mechanism, if not the site of the pain. The patient will generally want to describe what people said, what therapies they have had, and perhaps produce a pocket full of tablets. Worries and fears are usually revealed by sympathetic listening and these need resolving at the end of the consultation.

The present episode of back pain that brought Mr K.G., a 37 year old executive, to seek help started as a sharp pain in the lower back whilst stooping in his garden a month before. The next day he had to stay in bed because his back was so painful, and he had three days off work. After returning to the office, some back pain remained, but gradually over a second week it affected the left thigh and subsequently the left ankle. He came off work again, and was still troubled with pain in the left leg. Motivation was good; he would not be off work unless he was in considerable trouble. One would not be surprised to find marked restricted straight leg raising, and an acute disc prolapse.

Mr R.J. is 54 years old, has an unpleasant job in the coal mine, and six months ago he slipped underground on some wet sleepers. The water should not have been there and he describes the incident in great detail. He has not worked since. He did not have to go to bed, but rested at home, hoping the pain would settle. He complains aggressively of constant pain in the back and one thigh, and says he could not possibly manage his heavy underground job. He may have a genuine organic problem, but his failure to seek specialist help sooner, would make one suspicious about a non-organic element.

Mrs J.P. finds it difficult to identify when this present episode began. The back pain seems to have developed insidiously over the past year. She is 45 years old, overweight, and finds that her back aches after standing for long, shopping, and when rising from the stooping position. When it is particularly severe, it affects the upper thighs and she will lie down to obtain relief. One will be considering an instability type problem, and possibly isthmic or degenerative spondylolisthesis.

Mrs B.H. is 48 years of age, and for the first time developed pain in the right leg seven weeks ago. It was initially mild discomfort in the buttock and posterior thigh, but she continued her job as a teacher, stooping over small children at their desks. Three weeks ago the pain became very severe and it also affected the posterior calf and ankle. She is now off work and can find no relief from the pain. It keeps her awake at night, making her get up and walk about. She cannot sit or stand for long, and she keeps shuffling in the chair as she gives her history. Such a story is compatible with a root entrapment associated with degenerative changes in the root canal.

Mrs J.H. is 72 years old, and presents with a 10 week history of increasing upper lumbar pain, but no previous history of back pain. It is now constant and so severe that she spends much of the day lying down. Are these the first symptoms of spinal metastases?

Listening to the patient's story, with little prompting, will provide us with information often more valuable and more relevant than any examination or investigation. We learn much by listening. The very adjectives used to describe the intensity and character of the pain reflect the degree of distress. For some this is great and unfortunately we are least able to help by diagnosis and management, those who suffer most (Leavitt et al, 1979).

Childhood history

The childhood history can illuminate the present problem. It is worth asking if there was any violent injury in infancy or childhood. A quarter of patients with a lytic defect of the pars-interarticularis can remember some early injury such as a fall downstairs, a fall from a roof or a wall or out of a tree. The age of such an injury may relate to the degree of vertebral displacement, an injury in infancy permitting many years of growth to deform the vertebra, whilst an injury in late teens may disturb or initiate a spondylolysis without subsequent displacement. It would be helpful if enough clinicians recorded the method of birth of their patients with isthmic spondylolisthesis. It would refute or confirm the suggestion that birth injury can be responsible for lytic defects of the pars (Hitchcock, 1940, Rowe and

Roche, 1953). Our own small study of patients with defects suggests that there is a low incidence of Caesarean section in these patients.

Family history

In general a knowledge of the family history is unhelpful. Many patients will recount with enthusiasm a whole series of back pain sufferers within the family circle, but it has yet to be shown that inheritance is important. There is often a strong family history in dysplastic spondylolisthesis, and sometimes in isthmic spondylolisthesis. The influence of heredity on disc resiliance and on the vertebral canal configuration is yet unknown. The inherited HLA B-27 antigen increases the risk of developing ankylosing spondylitis but in general the family history is unhelpful.

Occupational history

The occupational history, however, is very relevant and deserves careful documentation. Spinal abuse in early adult life can be paid for dearly in later years. The middle aged housewife may have spent several years as a farm hand two decades before. The shopkeeper of today may have been yesterday's coal miner, tractor driver or bricklayer, now exhibiting spinal degenerative change. Wrestling, water ski-ing, parachute jumping are potentially hazardous pursuits with risk of back pain in later years. The price of a weak annulus and disc herniation may be a college education, a sedentary job, and then a single day's work in the garden.

Obstetric history

The obstetric history cannot be neglected, with instability problems beginning during pregnancy, delivery or in the puerperium. The joint laxity of pregnancy and the altered biomechanics can be risk factors heralding a chronic disability.

2. THE EXAMINATION

We like to think that the examination will produce objective data to formulate a diagnosis. In practice, it is more of a subjective assessment, though none the worse for that. There is a surprisingly high intra and inter-observer error in tests as simple as range of movement, or straight leg raising (Nelson et al, 1979, Waddell, 1982) but that does not invalidate the impressions these tests give to the clinician. A careful examination, though not necessarily highly repeatable, will provide the astute clinician with enough information to make his assessment about diagnosis and management. The examination began in fact, as the patient entered the consulting room. Was he limping, stooped, listing to one side, or walking with short steps? Whilst giving the history, much is revealed by the patient's attitude. We suspect the patient who tells a tale of woe with a smiling face; the obsessional patient who has written down a catalogue of symptoms; the depressed lacking facial expression; the hysteric indifferent to his symptoms, and the defensive or aggressive malingerer.

It is worth having a standard method of examination, one of which is described.

Look for spinal asymmetry and deformity. The commonest spinal deformity is a gravity induced list, occurring in 5 per cent of patients attending a back pain clinic (Porter and Miller, 1984). The centre of gravity is generally shifted to the left with the right hip prominent (66 per cent), less commonly to the right (31 per cent) and occasionally alternating from one side to the other (3 per cent) (Fig. 8.1). Remak first described the alternating list in 1891. The list is abolished by lying down and by hanging onto a bar. It can be apparently corrected when standing on the contra-lateral leg alone. It is almost pathognomonic of a disc lesion, and carries a relatively poor prognosis for conservative management but it gives no clue to the level of the lesion, its laterality or topographic position.

There are, of course, many other causes of a lumbar scoliosis. Structural scoliosis from morphological changes in the vertebrae is not corrected by lying down. Postural scoliosis compensates for a short leg and is simple to correct with a heel raise. Scoliosis secondary to spinal infection or tumour (Kirwan et al, 1984) must be considered when a list is unaltered by gravity.

Loss of lumbar lordosis may be associated with a disc lesion, or increased lordosis can compensate for an exaggerated thoracic kyphosis. Neither are corrected by lying down.

Look for two inappropriate signs in the standing

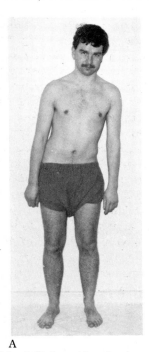 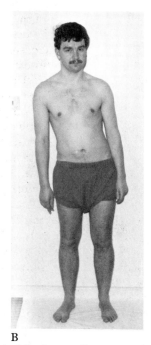 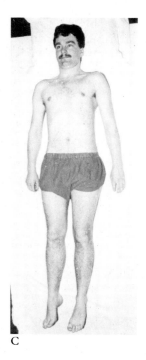

A   B   C

Fig. 8.1 A, Patient with an involuntary list to the left when standing.
B, He could change the list to the right at will.
C, The list was abolished by lying down. He subsequently had excision of an L.4/5 herniated disc.

patient; neither should be painful if the back pain has a mechanical origin. Apply vertical pressure to the skull. Is the axial loading painful? Then ask the patient to keep his feet immobile and rotate the pelvis on the lower limbs. Lumbar pain to simulated rotation should be regarded with suspicion.

Spinal mobility

How far can the patient bend forwards? To the floor, the upper tibiae, the mid thighs only? The ability to bend forwards is a combination of spinal and hip flexion, and is related more to good straight leg raising than to spinal flexion. Patients with an acute disc lesion may find it difficult to reach even to the knees. In contrast, those with isthmic or degenerative spondylolisthesis may easily place the flat of the hands on the floor, in spite of considerable back pain (Fig. 8.2).

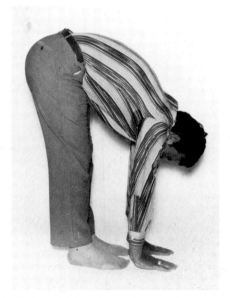

Fig. 8.2 Patient with isthmic spondylolisthesis and chronic low back pain, able to place the hands flat on the floor.

Mobility of the spine is usefully measured either with a tape-measure (Fig. 8.3) (Moll and Wright, 1971, Scott, 1983), or more rapidly and accurately with a goniometer (Loebl, 1967, and Reynolds, 1975) (Fig. 8.4).

Observe how the patient stands up again. Is the movement accomplished smoothly or with an extension catch? The catch is a jerky hesitancy half way through the process of standing up from the stooped position, and is a sign of spinal instability. Another instability sign (though sometimes seen in other back pain syndromes) is the necessity to use the hands to support the trunk by 'climbing up the legs' (Fig. 15.3).

Ask the patient to lean backwards, supporting the shoulders. An assessment of extension is highly subjective, but one gets an impression of loss of extension, to a third or two thirds of the normal range. Some patients, where space in the vertebral canal is at a premium, cannot even stand upright. They adopt a 'Simian' stance (Simkin, 1982, p. 111) with the hips and knees slightly flexed. They may temporarily force a more normal stance but will relapse again when distracted.

Lateral flexion is usually good in patients with lumbar pain of mechanical origin, and is equal on both sides unless there is a list. The patient with gross restriction of lateral flexion has other spinal or para spinal pathology, or perhaps a non organic lesion.

Assessment of the spine prone

Sacrospinalis hypertrophy is difficult to quantitate, but it sometimes accompanies instability, and is more easily detected with the patient prone (Fig. 8.5).

The spinous processes are identified by palpation. A list associated with a disc lesion will have corrected but not a structural scoliosis. Firm pressure on the spinous processes will reveal the level of the pain source. An L.4/5 disc can be very tender over L.4 and L.5 spinous processes; an L.5/S.1 disc over L.5. A patient who fractured the body of L.2 a year ago, and who is now tender over L.5 probably has lower lumbar pathology sustained at the same time and still a source of pain. One suspects upper lumbar pathology with lower lumbar pain if L.1 or L.2 is tender; the pain source is more likely to be in the upper lumbar spine with pain referred to the lower lumbar region. Root pain can occasionally be reproduced by maintained pressure on a spinous process, called by the French, a 'doorbell sign'.

Sacro-iliac tenderness is uncommon. Many patients have pain in the region of the sacro-iliac joints and to convince the clinician of its site, will confess to some tenderness. When specifically asked 'I know this is where you feel the pain, but I want to know if it is

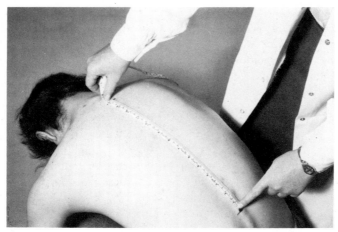

Fig. 8.3 The changing distance between two defined points, measured with a tape measure, provides an objective record of spinal mobility.

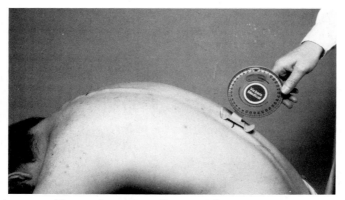

Fig. 8.4 Spinal range can be measured by a goniometer recording over defined fixed points.

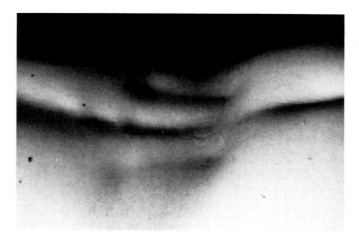

Fig. 8.5 Hypertrophied sacrospinal muscles of a 48 year old man, relaxed and lying prone. He had low back pain mainly standing and rising from the stooped position and had a degenerative spondylolisthesis at L.4/5.

tender', they generally confess the tenderness is over the lower lumbar spinous processes and not over the sacro iliac joints. Sacro iliac tenderness suggests either an inflammatory lesion of these joints, or of the soft tissues of the posterior pelvis.

Sacral tenderness should be regarded with suspicion. It is either a sinister sign of bony metastases, or a sign of an exaggerated response. Coccygeal tenderness is compatible with a recent history of trauma but if longstanding, it is probably inappropriate.

At this stage, gently squeeze the skin over the site of lumbar tenderness. If unduly painful, it is an inappropriate sign. The femoral stretch test is best

or girth to be objectively measured? Is there atrophy of the quadriceps or extensor digitorum brevis? There is no universal agreement about the correct way to perform the straight leg raising test. One method is to support the heel in the cupped hand of the examiner, and having explained the method to the patient, gently lift the heel from the couch with the knee still extended. The patient's head should be resting on one pillow and the arms relaxed by the side. The manoeuvre stops when the patient complains of pain, the angle is assessed and he is asked about the site of that pain. Crossed leg pain is pathognomonic of a disc lesion. Whilst holding the leg in this position, the foot is dorsiflexed to see if tension on the posterior tibial

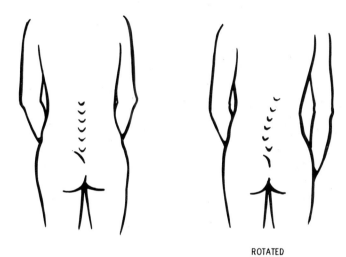

ROTATED

Fig. 8.6   Diagram to show that the floating segment of L.5 will remain a line with S.1 as the spine is rotated.

elicited with the patient prone. Flexing the knee alone will cause tension of the L.2 and L.3 roots, and may be sufficient to produce back pain. It will be increased by extending the hip. Pain arising in the hip is not influenced by flexing the knee alone. If lying prone is too painful, the tension signs can be tested with the patient on the side.

In this position, it is also possible to identify the floating segment of an isthmic spondylolisthesis. As the lumbar spine is rotated, the spinous process of a floating segment will fail to move. There is sequential lateral movement in an intact spine (Fig. 8.6).

Lower limbs supine

Look at the lower limbs. Is there asymmetry of length

nerve increases the sensation of pain (Bragaad's test). In the same position, the limb is externally rotated, relaxing the sacral plexus, and then internally rotated, increasing root tension; the experience of pain (Brieg & Troup, 1979) is recorded. At the limit of straight leg raising, the knee is first flexed and then extended, and the medial popliteal nerve compressed with the examining fingers of one hand, the 'Bow string test'. The Lasague test elicits pain in the leg or back, when at the limit of straight leg raising the knee is slightly flexed, the hip further flexed, and the knee then extended. These tension signs are generally present when a lower lumbar or sacral root is involved in the pathological process of pain. They are marked with acute root involvement from a disc protrusion, but mild or absent with nerve root irritation from long standing degenerative change.

Many patients are aware of the straight leg raising test, and for many reasons, conscious or unconscious, will influence its result. The examiner suspects voluntary resistance and can confirm this by combining the various stretch tests. He can flex the knee and record the range of hip flexion. If with the flexed knee the hip is limited in flexion, either there is hip pathology, or an exaggeration (though low back pain can at times be so severe that even flexing the hip aggravates the pain). Suspicions of exaggeration are confirmed, if on the pretext of examining the back, the patient is asked to sit up and lean forwards on the couch, and with extended knees he can reach well forwards to the feet. The 'Flip test' is similarly useful; when the knee of the seated patient is extended, he will 'flip over' backwards is straight leg raising is genuinely limited.

The Burn's test expects a patient to be able to kneel on a bench with knees and hips fully flexed, and place the fingers on the floor. Failure to do so is inappropriate and is said to correlate with hysteria on the MMPI (Evanski et al, 1979).

An inflammatory lesion of the sacro iliac joint is painful if the hip is flexed to ninety degrees and then forcibly adducted. This pain is, however, also experienced when there are positive root tension signs, and when there is an inflammatory lesion of the soft tissues of the posterior pelvis. Distraction of the pelvis, and compression on the anterior superior iliac spines, also aggravates sacro-iliac pain.

The knee and ankle reflexes should be symmetrical. Equal diminution is not significant, but asymmetrical reduction helps to identify an affected root. The knee reflex is usually subserved by the L.3, L.4 and L.5 roots, and the ankle reflex by the L.5 and S.1 roots.

The motor power of selected muscles is recorded EHL (S.1), Peronei (S.1), Quadriceps (L.4 and 5). Wasting of the quadriceps can be measured, and the Extensor Digitorum Brevis is a useful little muscle; its wasting can be observed and palpated in some S.1 root lesions. Weakness of the EHL is not uncommon but when other muscles are affected, there is either serious pathology or exaggeration. Weakness without wasting is highly suspect.

The sensation is recorded using a sharp pin. Numbness of the big toe (L.5) or of the outer foot (S.1) are encountered most frequently. A non dermatomal distribution is a useful observation, may be an inappropriate sign, but is highly subjective for both patient and doctor.

An extensor plantar reflex identifies an upper motor neurone lesion, which would be supported by brisk reflexes or clonus. Ataxia may have been suspected from the patient's gait, and confirmed by abnormal position sense of the big toe. If there is hesitancy, impaired proprioception will be supported by a tuning fork vibration test, and by asking the patient to run the heel of one foot down the opposite shin.

Palpate the dorsalis pedis and anterior tibial arteries, and if absent, check the femoral arteries in the groin. Is there a femoral bruit? An impaired peripheral circulation may explain the source of claudication pain, or it may co-exist with spinal pathology. One absent pulse may be irrelevant.

The examination is not complete without being sure that the hip and knee are not responsible for lower limb pain. Palpation of the abdomen is also mandatory. Occasionally an abdominal mass will explain the cause of pain.

We have mentioned many signs that would suggest an exaggerated response. Strange postures or abnormal gait, resisted movements, which change during the period of consultation, widespread and variable weakness with no muscle wasting, sweating and collapsing are inappropriate signs. It is useful to look specifically for six such signs (Waddell et al, 1980 and 1984). (Fig. 8.7):

1. Pain in the lumbar region when the skull is compressed vertically; axial loading.
2. Pain when the pelvis is rotated on the lower limbs whilst the patient is standing; simulated rotation.
3. Widespread tenderness.
4. Pain when the skin of the back is lightly squeezed.
5. Straight leg raising resisted voluntarily but improved with distraction.
6. Non dermatomal sensory reduction.

Their presence does not indicate the absence of an organic lesion, but it does make both the identification of that lesion more difficult, and its response to treatment disappointing. They are an exhibition of distress.

The history has provided the clinician with an

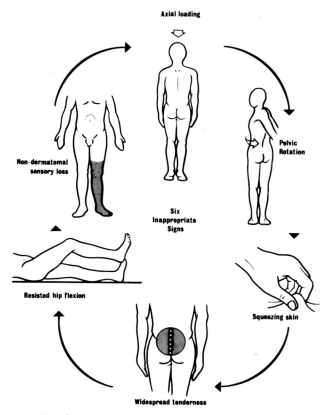

Axial loading

Pelvic Rotation

Non-dermatomal sensory loss

Six Inappropriate Signs

Resisted hip flexion

Squeezing skin

Widespread tenderness

Fig. 8.7   Diagrammatical representation of six inappropriate signs.

understanding of the patient's problem subjectively perceived, with its apparent dimensions in time, severity, and disability. The examination points to the diagnosis and helps to distinguish how much of the problem has a non organic element.

3. THE DISCUSSION

From the patient's position, this is the crux of the consultation. He wants to know if we have reached any conclusions about the cause of back pain, if any further tests are necessary, and what is needed to put things right. We probably err on the side of not talking enough to our patients. They want information. We should not withhold it. The first consultation is the ideal opportunity to explain the probable mechanism of the pain, and mismanagement now will compound problems which can be difficult to resolve.

The only investigation that is required for many patients with back pain is a plain radiograph, and if this has been performed previously, it allows the consultation to be completed at one sitting. If we have reached a presumptive diagnosis, it should be explained in simple terms, with a description of any necessary confirmatory tests. Methods of treatment or management and a word about prognosis puts the patient's mind at rest, and he should leave the consulting room in a lighter frame of mind.

4. INVESTIGATIONS

Investigations supplement, but are no substitute for a good history and examination. No single investigation will identify the source of back pain. We need to know the scope of each investigation, their indications, limitations and risks.

No assessment of a spine is complete without radiographs. There has been debate about their value and in isolation they are positively unhelpful. A report of radiographs describing perhaps degenerative changes or a spondylolisthesis, is irrelevant if divorced from the history and examination. In combination, however, they add valuable information and allow a rational approach to diagnosis and management (Chapter 9).

Haematological and Biochemical investigations will be required, if from the examination we suspect an inflammatory lesion or intra osseous pathology. It is not cost effective to screen every patient, nor indeed is it necessary. A raised erythrocyte sedimentation rate will support an inflammatory disorder, but it can be raised from many other unrelated conditions. A high E.S.R. may be associated with bony pathology, and if this is suspected, there is need for other blood tests, acid and alkaline phosphatase, serum proteins, and a differential white count. It may be necessary to examine the bone marrow, and test the urine for Benze-Jones protein. Gout can be an unsuspected diagnosis and not a few patients admitted with low back pain have a raised uric acid. Skeletal demineralisation requires estimation of serum calcium, phosphorus and alkaline phosphatase, and sometimes a bone biopsy to diagnose osteomalacia.

Only a few need further investigation. These are generally patients whose back pain is causing severe disability, and surgery is being considered.

Ultrasound Doppler scan is of particular value in the claudicating patient to assure us of the patency of the peripheral arteries. It is no more accurate than careful palpation, but a Doppler scan will give an objective record useful for the doubtful peripheral pulse, especially in the obese.

Ultrasound measurement of the vertebral canal adds a further dimension to the diagnostic quest. It is not an investigation that has gained widespread acceptance, and will probably not be generally used until improved imaging offers better results.

Nerve conduction tests will support a diagnosis of peripheral nerve entrapment of the lateral popliteal nerve at the neck of the fibula, and of the posterior tibial nerve in Tarsal Tunnel Syndrome. Unilateral delayed conduction and or reduced latency is a helpful sign.

Electromyographic studies will confirm the presence of impaired nerve function in the chronic but not the acute phase (Leyshon et al, 1980). Selective muscle degeneration can be identified and suggest the nerve root responsible but the root cannot be identified with complete confidence because of anomalies of nerve supply to individual muscles (Merriam et al, 1982). Electrical studies are useful in the patient who has exaggerated signs, and yet there is a possibility of genuine root pathology. Negative electro myographic findings do not exclude genuine symptoms but positive results confirm significant root damage.

Thermography, being non-invasive, is an attractive investigation if it can be confidently interpreted. Methods employing crystalography will record skin temperature changes in the order of half a degree centigrade. It can provide objective evidence of pain sensation, because the skin overlying an area of pain is cooler than its contralateral area. It is probably an unnecessary investigation for the clinician who is assured of his own assessment of the patient, but it is an attractive objective test. Its role in the management of back pain is not yet established.

Further radiographs especially with contrast radiography are indicated when surgery is a serious possibility. Metrizamide radiculography is the investigation of choice, and other secondary contrast techniques depend on the experience of the radiologist.

Spinal scintigraphy helps to diagnose facet fracture, stress fracture of the pars, and acute disruption of an existing pars defect. It is of more value than radiography in the early diagnosis of sacroiliitis and of spinal tumour or infection.

CT has now revolutionised spinal imaging. It compets with radiculography for the initial test. It has expanded the horizons of the clinician, offering information about the hidden areas of the spine, the vertebral canal, its size and shape. It demonstrates the degree and extent of stenosis, and soft tissue involvement. It provides valuable information about the post-operative spine. Its biggest demand is probably for the detection and assessment of disc disorders. The patient is spared the morbidity of radiculography, and the cost is not dissimilar to that of a contrast study. When the CT findings are inconclusive, or do not explain the clinical features, it is then helpful to perform radiculography and repeat the CT study whilst the contrast medium is still present (Anad and Lee, 1982).

Nuclear magnetic resonance has yet to come of age and find its place in spinal investigations. An absence of fat may support central canal stenosis or lateral stenosis, and it may help to identify spinal cord trauma and spinal infection. Disc degeneration is easily visualised, but not protrusion (Modic et al, 1983).

The expansion of investigative techniques can be counter-productive if it outstrips our skill in taking the patient's history and performing a good examination. These are paramount, and any gross pathology we may identify by sophisticated investigation has little value unless it corresponds with the patient's symptomatology.

In addition, we should pause to question what is to be gained by exposing our patients to high powered technology, when our therapeutic skills have not kept pace with improved investigations. Investigation is of value only if it affects that patient's management.

REFERENCES

Anad A K, Lee B C 1982 Plain and metrizamide CT of lumbar disc disease. American Journal of Neuroradiology 3: 567–571

Breig A, Troup J D G 1979 Biomechanical considerations in the straight leg raising test. Spine 4: 242–250

Evanski P M, Carver D, Nehemkis A, Waugh T R, 1979 The Burn's test in low back pain. Clinical Orthopaedics and Related Research 140: 42–44

Hitchcock H H 1940 Spondylolisthesis. Journal of Bone and Joint Surgery 22: 1–16

Kirwan E O'G, Hutton P A N, Pozo J L, Ransford A O 1984 Osteoid osteoma and benign osteoblastoma of the spine: clinical presentation and treatment. Journal of Bone and Joint Surgery 66–B: 21–26

Leavitt F, Garron D C, D'Angelo C M, McNeill T W 1979 Low back pain in patients with or without demonstrable organic disease. Pain 6: 191–200

Leyshon A, Kirwan E O'G, Wynn Parry C B 1980 Is it nerve root pain? Journal of Bone and Joint Surgery 62–B: 119

Loebl W Y 1967 Measurement of spinal posture and range of spinal movement. Annals of Physical Medicine 9: 103–110

McGee A 1961 The patient's attitude to nursing care. Edinburgh: Livingstone

Merriam W F, Smith N J, Mulholland R C 1982 Lumbar spinal stenosis. British Medical Journal 285: 515

Modic M T, Weinstein M A, Pavlicek W et al 1983 Nuclear Magnetic resonance imaging of the spine. Radiology 148: 757–762

Moll J M H, Wright V 1971 Normal range of spinal mobility: an objective clinical study. Annals of Rheumatology 30: 381–386

Nelson M A, Allen P, Clamp S E, de Dombal F T 1979 Reliability and reproducibility of clinical findings in low back pain. Spine 4: 97–101

Porter R W and Miller C 1984. Gravity induced list. Presented to the International Society for the Study of the Lumbar Spine, Montreal. Remak E 1891 Deutsch Med Woch 257

Reynolds P M G 1975 Measurement of spinal mobility: a comparison of three methods. Rheumatology and Rehabilitation 14: 180–185

Rowe G G, Roche M B 1953 The aetiology of separate neural arch. Journal of Bone and Joint Surgery, 35–A: 102–110

Scott J H S 1983 Clinical examination. Sixth Edition Churchill Livingstone, Edinburgh London Melbourne and New York

Simkin P A 1982 Simian stance: a sign of spinal stenosis. The Lancet 652–653

Waddell G 1982 An approach to backache. British Journal of Hospital Medicine. September

Waddell G, McCulloch J A, Kummell E and Venner R M 1980 Nonorganic physical signs in low back pain. Spine 5: 117–125

Waddell G, Main C J, Morris E W, Di Paola M and Gray I C M 1984 Chronic low back pain. Psychological Distress and Illness Behaviour. Spine 9: 209–213

Wright V, Hopkins R, Burton K 1982 How long should we talk to patients? A study in doctor-patient communication. Annals of the Rheumatic Diseases 41: 250–252

9

Radiographic investigation of back pain

There is a dilemma about the clinical value of radiological investigation. Plain radiography shows but shadows of the bones, leaving us to guess the condition of the more important soft structures. Gross disability can accompany normal films, and normal spinal function is compatible with marked degenerative change. It is not surprising, therefore, that radiologists can make little sense of films divorced from the real patient, and clinicians examining patients cannot rely on reported films. Curry et al (1979) suggests that lumbar radiographs should be reserved for the back pain problem that fails to settle speedily.

In spite of these reservations about the value of lumbar radiographs, if the films are of good quality, are carefully examined and matched with a good history and clinical examination, they undoubtedly are the most useful single investigation available to the clinician.

1. PLAIN RADIOGRAPHS

Ageing has an important effect on the spine, and degenerative changes can be expected at the lower lumbar levels in 95 per cent of both sexes by 70 years of age. The rate at which this occurs is so variable that it is difficult to distinguish 'premature' disc degeneration from the effects of age (Park 1980). The presence of intranuclear gas — the so called 'vacuum phenomenon' — is a radiological sign associated with a cleft or fissure in the annulus fibrosus. When structural failure of the disc occurs, the radiological effect is to produce disc space narrowing, with reactive sclerosis of the adjacent vertebral bone (Fig. 9.1).

Osteophytes can give a clue to what is happening to the disc, but not with total reliability. Traction spurs

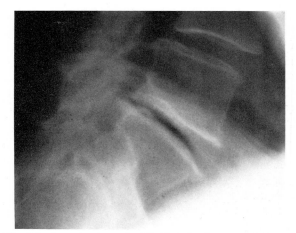

Fig. 9.1 Lateral radiograph of L.5/S.1 showing signs of disc degeneration — a 'vacuum phenomenon', disc space narrowing, and reactive sclerosis.

are usually associated with disc degeneration (Quinnell and Stockdale, 1982). They develop a few millimeters from the upper and lower borders of the vertebral bodies, grow into the attachments of the anterior longitudinal ligament and annular fibres, and are generally accepted as a sign of instability (Fig. 3.4, page 16). Claw-type osteophytes develop at the very edge of the vertebral body margin around the annulus, and they may meet and fuse the two vertebrae together. They may be associated with disc degeneration, but are quite compatible with a normal discogram (Fig. 3.3, page 15).

Although the disc has a structure of key importance in the spine, it is unusual to find degenerative change at the disc space alone. Schmorl and Junghanns (1971) used the term 'motor segment' to include all the supportive tissues that span each disc-apophyseal joint complex, and when the disc fails, it also involves this segmental complex. The apophyseal joints are usually involved but are not easy to visualise. If degenerative change cannot be seen on standard radiographs, axial views are required. The articular surface presents itself tangentially to the x-ray beam only in one plane, and with the joint orientation gradually and sequentially changing from the sagittal to coronal plane proximo-distally, the joints of the whole lumbar spine can never be seen on one film. Osteophytic outgrowths from the apophyseal joints not only restrict movements but can compromise the root canal, especially by reactive proliferation of capsular and other soft tissues overlying the apophyseal osteophytes. The combined changes can be clinically significant if that canal is already narrowed or trefoil in shape, or if there is a prolapsed intervertebral disc.

Isthmic spondylolisthesis is usually suspected from the lateral and antero-posterior radiograph. It is conventional to grade the severity of olisthesis by the amount of forward displacement over the sacrum. On the lateral film, the disc surface of the sacrum is arbitrarily divided into quarter segments. Grades 1 to 4 are used to represent the position of the displaced vertebra in relation to these quarters. Alternatively, the 'slip-ratio' is the percentage forward displacement of the posterior border of the proximal vertebral body (Fig. 9.2).

With a lysis at L.5 the body is usually wedged, more so with greater displacement. A shelf of anterior sacral prominence has usually developed in an attempt to stabilise the listhesis. These changes develop during the period of growth, and are sometimes of such degree that ossification completely stabilises the segment (Fig. 9.3).

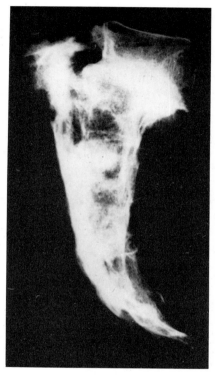

Fig. 9.3   Radiographic specimen of isthmic spondylolisthesis at L.5/S.1 stabilised by spontaneous bony fusion.

In the antero-posterior view, spondylolisthesis may be suspected from the apparent density of the tilted lamina. If the defect in the pars interarticularis is not evident in the lateral projection, then oblique views give the classically described 'Scottie dog collar' (Fig. 9.4). A unilateral defect may only be displayed by a 45 degree oblique angle, inclined cranially at 20 degrees.

It is difficult to measure the sagittal diameter of the vertebral canal from a lateral radiograph. Eisenstein (1977) suggested that the translucency at the base of the spinous process represents the posterior margin of the canal, but this is rarely seen when it matters, in patients with degenerate narrow canals. However, the

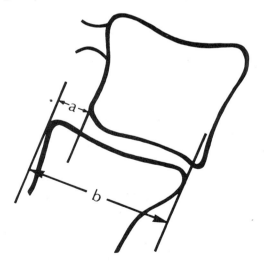

$$\frac{a}{b} \times 100 = \text{Slip ratio}$$

Fig. 9.2   Method of measuring the slip ratio.

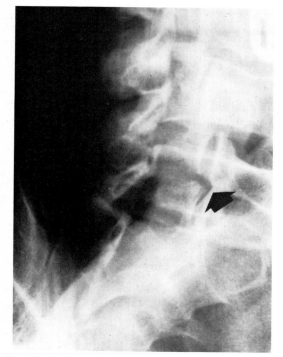

Fig. 9.4 45 degree oblique radiograph showing a pars defect at L.5, the 'scottie dog collar'.

lateral view frequently gives an impression of the canal's capacity.

Flexion and extension views are sometimes helpful in a patient with instability symptoms and when posture affects root pain. They can demonstrate horizontal shear or excessive intervertebral tilt. This unnatural segmental movement can be the result of disc degeneration (Fig. 9.5) or be secondary hypermobility distal to a congenital block vertebra (Fig. 9.6) or adjacent to a surgical fusion. It may, of course, be symptomless.

Miscellaneous conditions

A variety of miscellaneous conditions can be recognised from plain radiographs of the lumbar spine. They may reveal a fracture of the vertebral body or neural arch, suspected after significant trauma. The diagnosis of vertebral osteomyelitis can be made with confidence, in the presence of gross end-plate destruction, disc space narrowing and paravertebral abscess. Tuberculosis, though rare, may be overlooked unless suspicion is high. Its radiological features can, on occasion, be mistaken for

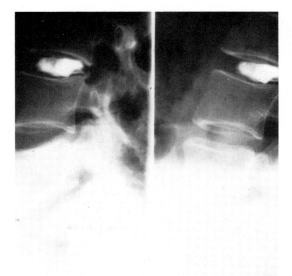

A

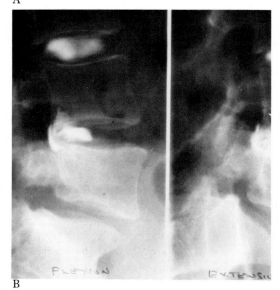

B

Fig. 9.5 A, Lateral radiograph in extension (left) and flexion (right) of a patient with isthmic spondylolisthesis at L.5/S.1, a discogram at L.3/4, and signs of excessive spinal movement at L.4/5
B, A discogram at L.4/5 of the same patient, showing a degenerate disc with disruption of the posterior annulus

degenerative disc disease. Relatively mild presentation of tuberculosis sometimes causes delay in diagnosis (Enarson et al, 1979).

The cancellous bone of the spine is a common site for metastases. The infiltrative process is manifest by destruction on the vertebral body leading to collapse. Metastatic destruction of the pedicles distinguishes

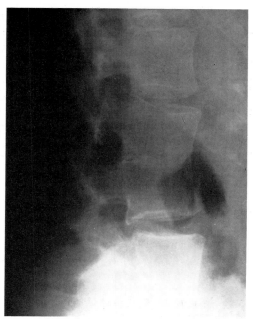

Fig. 9.6 Lateral radiograph showing a congenital block vertebra at L.3/4 with unnatural segmental movement at L.4/5

this from multiple myeloma. Diffuse irregular osteosclerosis is usually a sign of osteoblastic secondary deposits from breast cancer in women and from the prostate in men.

The spine is a rare site for primary neoplasm, but some tumours like osoteogenic sarcoma will give a characteristic appearance. Primary tumours, which may arise in the neural arch or pedicles, are osteoid osteoma, osteoblastoma, and aneurysmal bone cyst (page 7).

Paget's disease causes expansion and disorganisation on the bone with characteristic radiological appearances. It is often insidious and asymptomatic, and found incidentally with other bone involvement. It can cause cauda equina ischaemia and radiculopathy even in the presence of an adequate vertebral canal, though limited space from neural arch thickening, fracture or sarcomatous change can add to the problem.

Ankylosing spondylitis produces characteristic radiological changes in the spine and sacro-iliac joints, though sacroiliitis may not be obvious radiologically for a year or so after the onset of the illness. Radioscintigraphy with bone-seeking isotopes is more helpful for early diagnosis of sacroiliitis. The inflammatory process involves the vertebral end-

plates, squaring the margins of the vertebral bodies giving the appearance of 'discitis', and then intervertebral ossification with the painless 'bamboo spine'. Symptoms at this stage may herald secondary fracture or pseudoarthrosis.

A central Schmorl's node from disc herniation through the vertebral end-plate, is a frequent incidental finding on a lateral lumbar radiograph. An anterior node may follow trauma in childhood, and separate the ring epiphysis. The radiological appearance of Scheuermann's disease is quite characteristic. The upper lumbar vertebrae can be affected, though the thoracic spine is the commonest region of involvement. When advanced, there can be severe vertebral wedging, irregularity of vertebral end-plates, and multiple Schmorl's nodes.

30 per cent bone loss takes place before demineralisation is apparent radiologically. Severe osteoporosis produces the effect of ballooning of the discs with the increased biconcavity of the vertebral bodies giving the 'cod fish' appearance (Resnick, 1982). Wedging is frequent, from collapse compression fracture. The discs may calcify, which as an isolated finding is not of significance. General disc calcification however may accompany hyperparathyroidism, fluorosis, chondrocalcinosis and haemochromatosis.

2. CONTRAST RADIOGRAPHY

Metrizamide radiculography

This is usually the contrast study of choice to demonstrate a lesion or lesions affecting the nerve root, cauda equina or spinal cord. It is generally reserved for those patients considered suitable for surgery, a very small proportion of back pain sufferers. The decision to operate is based on clinical factors, but the radiologist can contribute by precise definition of site, extent and nature of the pathology. This information may influence the surgical approach and the most appropriate operation. A radiculogram using water-soluble contrast medium offers the most complete demonstration of the dural tube and its contents in the lower dorsal and lumbar regions. Metrizamide has proved highly satisfactory (Grainger et al, 1976), with only minor side effects of headache, nausea and vomiting though for a few patients this is distressing. It can persist if surgery follows quickly upon the radiculogram (Lynch and Dickson, 1983).

There have been no reports of adhesive arachnoiditis after using Metrizamide.

The demonstration of a posterior disc protrusion depends on obliteration of the nerve root cuff or a dural deformity. There are few false positives, but sensitivity is better at L.4/5 than L.5/S.1. Inability to demonstrate some lumbosacral disc lesions results from the occasional failure of dural sheaths to extend to this level. Similarly, in patients with root entrapment syndrome, where root canal stenosis affects the root distally, radiculography is usually of little help (Euinton et al, 1984).

Myelography is diagnostic in patients with neurogenic claudication where there may be one or several segment encroachment into a developmentally shallow vertebral canal. In general terms, an assessment of the degree of restriction of dural capacity can be made from the height of the contrast column when a fixed volume injection is made. Since the segmental defects are usually maximal in the erect or hyper-extended positions, flexion and extension films are recorded (Fig. 15.5, page 126).

Radiculography should be a standard procedure before spinal surgery. It will occasionally demonstrate an unsuspected but significant lesion (Fig. 9.7).

A negative or equivocal radiculogram, in the presence of strong clinical evidence of prolapsed intervertebral disc, may require additional investigation. It is clear that the most successful results of surgery are to be expected from a single, definitive procedure, and no price is too great to be sure of the pain source before operation. Disco-

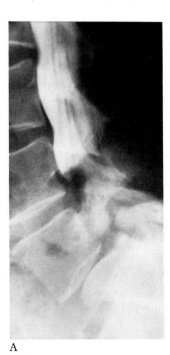
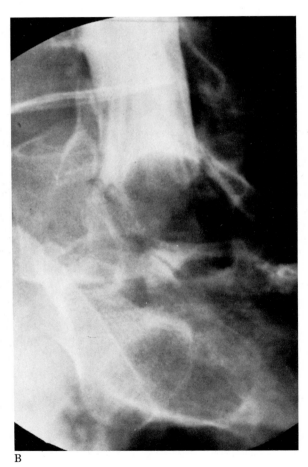

A   B

Fig. 9.7 A, Radioculogram prior to a proposed fusion for a 37 year old woman with severe low back pain and an isthmic spondylolisthesis
B, The well circumscribed filling defect proved to be a rare para ganglionoma.

graphy, epidural venography, epidurography or CT scan may be of help.

Discography

'Discography' was first introduced by Lindblohm (1948), who demonstrated the morphology of the nucleus pulposus by injecting contrast medium. The lateral approach is preferable. The amount of injection pressure required to fill the nucleus depends on the state of the disc. A normal nucleus has a characteristic resistance to injection, and can usually be delineated satisfactorily with 0.5 ml of contrast medium. The grossly degenerate disc, especially with an annular tear, has virtually no limit to the volume that can be injected.

Patients may experience pain during discography, which can help in identification of a symptomatic disc. This should be interpreted with caution however, because provocation of the sensitive annulus by needle penetration, or false injection into the annulus, can produce pain which may not be related in any way to the patient's symptoms.

The radiological appearances of normal and degenerate discs are quite characteristic. The outline of the degenerate nucleus is irregular, sometimes with a 'tissue sequestrum' filling defect and extravasation of the contrast medium (Fig. 9.5). A degenerate disc is not necessarily the seat of pain.

The diagnostic accuracy of lumbar discography was reviewed by Hudgins (1977) with a rate of 17 per cent false negatives, and 22 per cent false positives.

The relevance of discography is still the subject of some controversy, but it is undoubtedly useful precedeing chemonucleolysis and as a means of ensuring the integrity of the disc space proximal to a proposed fusion. It may be superseded by NMR.

Epidural venography

The technique requires some experience, and for this reason, epidural venography has not gained universal acceptance as a routine method of investigating the spine. It is particularly useful as a second contrast technique to demonstrate an extra-dural lesion that does not encroach on the dural sac, such as a postero-lateral disc at L.5/S.1. Venography can be superior in spinal stenosis, confirming its extent when myelography is technically difficult (Ehni, 1969,

Williams, 1975, Bestawros et al, 1979, Herkowitz et al, 1982).

Epidurography

Epidurography is not widely practised because of the toxicity of the ionic water-soluble contrast medium, should it be inadvertently introduced into the subarachnoid space (Nagamine, 1970). The sacral route is probably safer, but there is a danger of puncturing the epidural venous plexus. It does allow outline of the external surface of the dura and its extensions along the nerve roots, and will therefore identify pathology in areas not visualised by intrathecal contrast medium. It can be managed on an out-patient basis. It is not a practical procedure in post-laminectomy syndromes, when adhesive arachnoiditis distorts the epidural space.

Facet arthrography

Interest has focused on the apophyseal joints as a source of back and leg pain since Putti (1927) suggested that sciatica was commonly caused by vertebral arthritis. Ghormley (1933) introduced the term 'facet syndrome' to include patients with back pain only.

There is no doubt that these joints can be a source of pain. McCall et al (1979) provocatively injected 0.2–0.4 ml of hypertonic saline into the apophyseal joints of volunteers, and recorded a feeling of deep ache or cramp on the ipsilateral side at some distance from the injection sites, but never below the knee. How frequently the facet joints are a primary source of pain is open to question, though it is widely accepted that they frequently affect the nerve root in the root canal from osteophytic encroachment and capsular thickening (Epstein et al, 1973).

The recent enthusiasm for denervation of the apophyseal joints requires expertise in their visualisation by arthrography. The rationale, however, depends on accepting that they are a significant primary pain source, and this has yet to be proven.

Kellgren (1977) observed that experimental injection of 0.5 ml Methylene Blue stained a muscle mass of 6 cm, indicating a wide diffusion into the soft tissues. It would seem, therefore, that even if a needle is introduced accurately into the joint, interpretation of the effects of local anaesthetic is difficult because of the diffusion into surrounding tissues, especially to the root in the adjacent root canal.

Arthrography is easily performed in the x-ray department, with the patient prone, using a 9 cm needle (21G) directed obliquely downwards to the joint. The position of skin puncture depends on the orientation of the facets, and its direction is guided by television control. A sudden drop in resistance is felt as the joint is penetrated. 0.5 to 1 ml of contract will outline each joint.

Sometimes the apophyseal joints at two levels will communicate via the pars interarticularis and there may be fairly wide extensions of a hemi-sacralised unilateral articulation (Fig. 9.8). Whether or not a hemi-sacralised joint is a pain source is open to question.

As with all clinical investigations, the benefits have to be balanced against patient discomfort, complications and costs. Progress in the management of back pain will come through improved methods of diagnosis; that is improving our clinical assessment, and selecting the place of the best additional procedures to identify the lesion or lesions giving rise to pain.

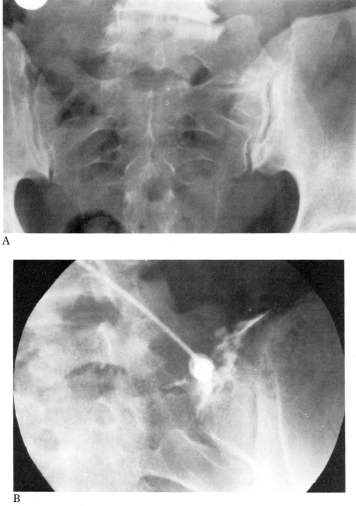

A

B

Fig. 9.8 A, Left sided hemi-sacralised L.5 with degenerative changes of the sacro iliac joint.
B, arthrography showing wide extension of the hemisacralised joint (by kind permission of Dr T Hughes).

REFERENCES

Bestawros O A, Vreeland O H, Golman M L 1979 Epidural venography in the diagnosis of lumbar spinal stenosis. Radiology 131: 423–426

Curry H L F, Greenwood R M, Lloyd G G, Murray R S 1979 A prospective study of low back pain. Rheumatology and Rehabilitation 18: 94–104

Ehni G 1969 Significance of the small lumbar spinal canal cauda equina compression syndromes due to spondylosis. Journal of Neurosurgery 31: 490–494

Eisenstein S 1977 Morphometry and pathological anatomy of the lumbar spine in South African negroes and caucasoids with specific reference to spinal stenosis. Journal of Bone and Joint Surgery 59–B: 173–180

Enarson D A, Fujii M, Nakielna E M, Grzybowski S 1979 Bone and joint tuberculosis; a continuing problem. Canadian Medical Association Journal 120: 139–145

Epstein J A, Epstein B S, Lavine L S, Carrass R, Rosenthal A D, Sumner P 1973 Lumbar nerve root compression at the intervertebral foramina caused by arthritis of the posterior facets. Journal of Neurosurgery 39: 362–369

Euinton H A, Locke T J, Barrington N A and Davies G K 1984. Radiological diagnosis of bony entrapment of lumbar nerve roots using water soluble radiculography. Presented to the International Society for Study of the Lumbar Spine, Montreal.

Ghormley R K 1933 Low back pain: with special reference to the articular facets, with presentation of an operative procedure. Journal of the American Medical Association 101: 1773–1777

Grainger R G, Kendall B E, Wylie I G 1976 Lumbar myelography with metrizamide — a new non-ionic contrast medium. British Journal of Radiology 49: 996–1003

Herkowitz H N, Weise I S W, Booth R E, Rothman R H 1982 Metrizamide myelography and epidural venography. Their role in the diagnosis of lumbar disc herniation and spinal stenosis. Spine 7: 55–64

Hudgins W R 1977 Diagnostic accuracy of lumbar discography. Spine 2 (4): 305–309

Kellgren J H 1977 The anatomical source of back pain. Rheumatology Rehabilitation 16: 7

Lindblohm K 1948 Diagnostic puncture of intervertebral discs in sciatica. Acta Orthopaedica Scandinavica 17: 231–239

Lynch A F, Dickson R A 1983 The relationship of complications to the time between myelography and discectomy. Journal of Bone and Joint Surgery 65–B: 259–261

McCall I W, Park W M, O'Brien J P 1979 Induced pain referral from posterior lumbar elements in normal subjects. Spine 4: 441–446

Nagamine K 1970 Clinical and biochemical study of accidents and peridurography. Nagoya Journal of Medical Science 32: 429–444

Park W M 1980 Radiology in the investigation of low back pain. Clinics in Rheumatic Diseases 6: 93–132

Putti V 1927 Lady Jones lecture on new conceptions in the pathogenesis of sciatic pain. Delivered at the University of Liverpool March 10th. Lancet ii, 53–60

Quinnell R C, Stockdale H R 1982 The significance of osteophytes on the lumbar vertebral bodies in relation to discographic findings. Clinical Radiology 23: 197–203

Resnick D L 1982 Fish vertebrae. Arthritis and Rheumatism 25: 1073–1077

Schmorl G, Junghanns H 1971 The human spine in health and disease. 2nd American Edition. New York Grune and Strathon

Williams R W 1975 The narrow lumbar spinal canal. Australasian Radiology 19, 356–360

The place of C.T. scanning in the investigation of back pain

One is rightly awed by the complexity of the computerised tomographic scanner and by the genius of its inventor. It is difficult not to let this influence one's assessment of its diagnostic accuracy and its place in the investigation of back pain. CT scanning, like all diagnostic radiology, is a demonstration of two-dimensional gross pathology in black, white and shades of grey but there is no inherent reason why a diagnosis demonstrated by a computer should be more accurate than a diagnosis demonstrated by shadows.

The pictures produced by the CT scanner are not images in the sense of shadows but are pictures of the mathematical solutions of n + 1 equations containing n unknowns. By assigning a shade of grey to a number, the scanner produces a black and white picture in which the anatomical structures are demonstrated in shades of grey depending on their radiation absorption. Currently, the apparatus has 2000 recordable stages between full black and full white and theoretically has incredible sensitivity in tissue differentiation. The assigned numbers can be manipulated mathematically to alter the contrast between structures, and measure distances, area, volume and radiation absorption of individual tissues. The more sophisticated apparatus can enhance edge contrast and manipulate the stored information to produce pictures in planes which were not part of the original radiographic exposure. The manipulations seem limited only by the imagination of the soft ware technicians.

The currently available apparatus has serious physical limitations in that the diameter of the central hole through which the patient must pass restricts many of the positions which are suitable for spinal assessment (Fig. 10.1). This, combined with the limitations of gantry angulation to plus or minus 20

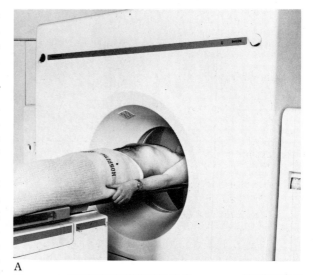

A

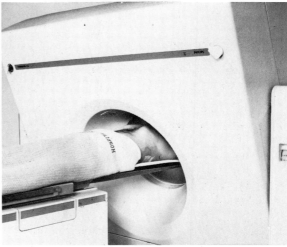

B

Fig. 10.1 (a). Pictures of a CT scanner demonstrates just how little room there is, b). Even with the gantry tilted some projections of the spine are impossible.

degrees, can prevent accurate demonstration of entities such as spondylolisthesis. The sensors are limited in size, and discrimination below 1 mm is, at the moment, unreliable. This compares unfavourably with standard radiographs which can define 5 or 6 line pairs per mm.

The radiographic beam used to obtain each CT scan is tightly collimated and the overall radiation dose during the examination is very similar to the radiation dose of a standard radiographic examination using the same factors. In practical terms, CT examination of the lumbar spine gives approximately twice the radiation dose of a routine radiographic examination.

APPLICATIONS OF THE CT SCANNER

Robinson (1983) has outlined the general applications of CT scanning:

1. To demonstrate areas not demonstrable by other techniques
2. To demonstrate normal anatomy
3. To make specific diagnoses
4. To assist and avoid invasive procedures
5. To assess the extent of disease
6. To monitor the effects of treatment.

It is particularly valuable in spinal investigation because it can produce a supero-inferior radiograph and it can differentiate tissues.

SUPERO-INFERIOR VIEW

1. Answers questions posed by frontal and lateral radiographs

This is the most practical and valuable contribution that CT scanning makes to the patient with back pain, (Haughton 1983). It is illustrated by the following examples.

A young adult woman with isthmic spondylolisthesis develops signs and symptoms of nerve root pathology. If a disc herniation is responsible it is usually at the level above the spondylolisthesis since the slip increases the space available for the nerve roots in the vertebral canal at the level of displacement. The routine myelographic examination revealed evidence of nerve root involvement but was not able to demonstrate the cause. The anatomical

deformity of spondylolisthesis is so great that the region is not easily demonstrated on standard radiographic projections, and even a 45 degree inclined frontal film in this patient did not reveal the cause of the root compression (Fig. 10.2). The CT scan shows root involvement by a displaced bifid posterior arch and not by the expected disc hernia.

Progressive kyphos of the dorsal spine associated with paraplegia is an uncommon but important clinical situation and in these patients the spinal deformity is often so great as to defy standard radiographic assessment. The supero-inferior radiographic facility of CT scanning allows us to distinguish patients with compression of the cord due simply to the kyphos (Fig. 10.3), patients with no abnormality of the kyphos (Fig. 10.4) and patients with direct cord compression from a lesion posteriorly at the kyphos (Fig. 10.5). This pre-operation assessment is essential for correct clinical management.

The grotesquely deformed spine which occurs with neurofibromatosis is often associated with unpredictable abnormalities. Fig. 10.6 demonstrates the myelographic appearance of a patient with neurofibromatosis and incipient paraplegia. The numerous indentations of the dorsal subarachnoid space were thought to be due to neurofibromatas until the CT scan demonstrated that the indentations were intraspinal herniations of the ribs in the region. Grotesque and unpredictable skeletal deformities are not uncommon with neurofibromatosis.

2. Demonstrates Areas not previously demonstrable on standard radiographic studies

Soft tissue encroachment into the root canal cannot be demonstrated on standard radiographic examination because the nerve root sleeves as demonstrated by myelography do not routinely fill to the entrance of these tunnels let alone throughout their length. This radiological blind spot is well demonstrated by CT (Fig. 10.7). Previous techniques such as nerve sheath injection and intra-osseous vertebral venography attempt to overcome this difficulty but have been surpassed by CT scanning. Those scanners which permit oblique reconstruction along the path of the root canal show the area to advantage, (Dorwart and Genant, 1983).

One of the common situations in which the facility

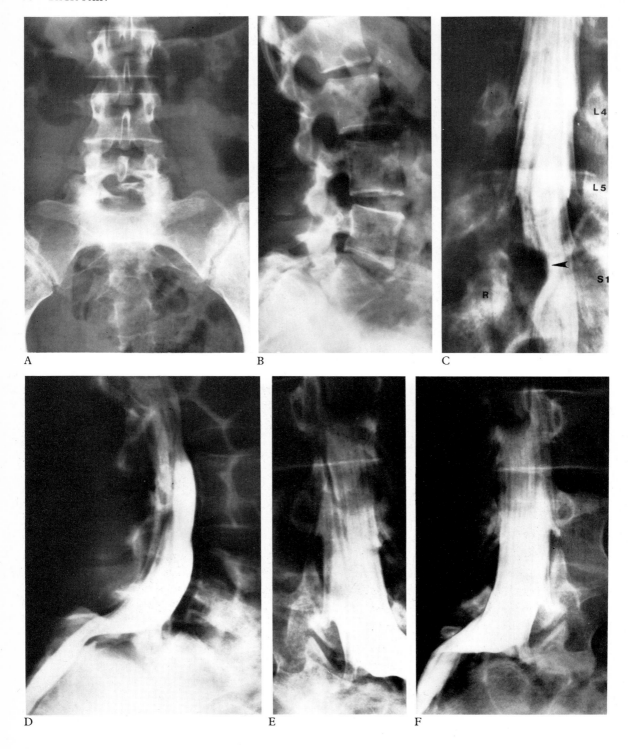

A

B

C

D

E

F

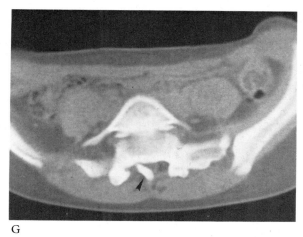

G

Fig. 10.2 (a, b, c, d, e, f, g). A series of films demonstrate the use of CT scanning in the assessment of the patient with spondylolisthesis and root pain. The nerve root compression (c) is not due to the anticipated disc hernia but rather to a rotated and displaced, bifid, posterior arch (g).

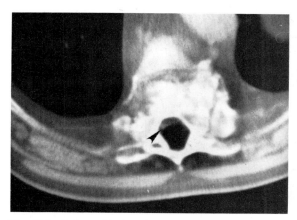

Fig. 10.3 Patient with thoracic kyphos and progressive paraplegia that demonstrates the value of CT in establishing the cause. Spinal cord traction by the kyphos.

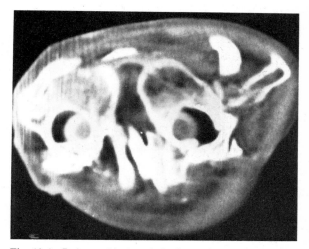

Fig. 10.4 Patient with thoracic kyphos and progressive paraplegia that demonstrates the value of CT in establishing the cause. No lesion near the kyphos.

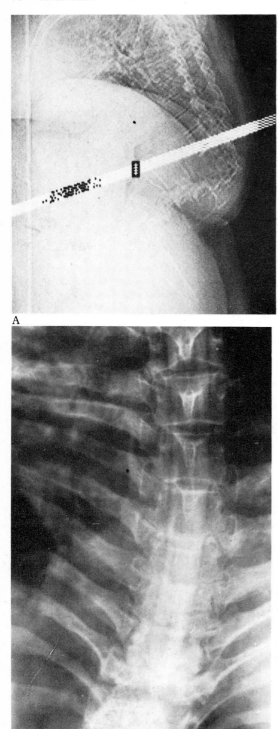

C

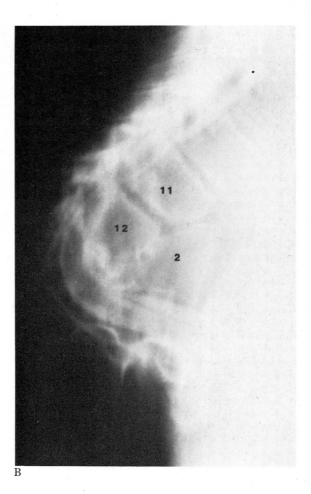

B

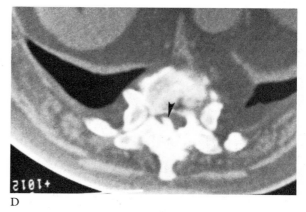

D

Fig. 10.5 Patients with thoracic kyphos and progressive paraplegia that demonstrates the value of CT in establishing the cause. Cord compression unrelated to the kyphos.
These last three figures demonstrate that which is not recognised by standard radiographs.

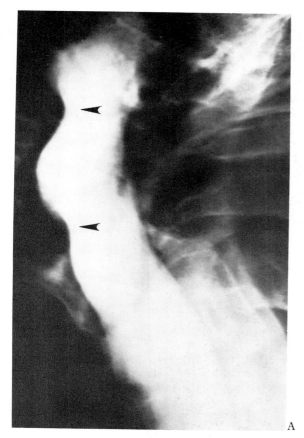

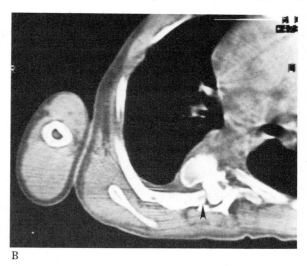

A

B

Fig. 10.6 Numerous indentations of the dye filled subarachnoid space (A) were thought to be due to neurofibromata but were shown, by CT scanning (B), to be due to impressions from herniated ribs. Unanticipated abnormalities are frequent in patients with neurofibromatosis. (Published with kind permission of Harper and Row Inc. 1984).

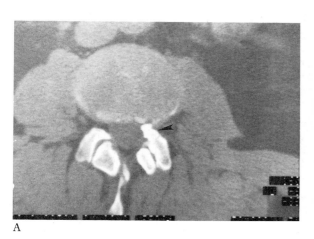

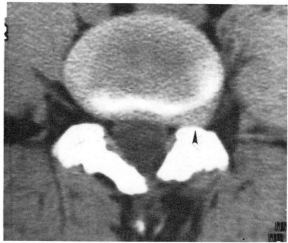

A   B

Fig. 10.7 CT scan showing the root canal compromised by (a) bony encroachment and (b) disc herniation

to demonstrate lateral encroachment on nerve roots is valuable occurs in patients with spondylolisthesis and root pain. A cartilaginous and/or ossified cuff will develop around a lysis of the pars interarticularis and on occasion this cuff can be large enough to compress the nerve root in the canal. This nerve root compression is almost invariably too far lateral to be demonstrated on a myelogram. Reliable demonstration of the level of the lesion is important because it affects the same nerve root at the lysis that would be compressed by a disc hernia at the level above, and clinical localisation is not, therefore possible. Figure 10.8 shows several examples of chondrified and ossified cuffs around spondylolyses.

Certain encroachments on the central vertebral canal occur in planes that are not amenable to standard radiography. One of these is circumferential thickening of the lamina in patients with previous inter-lamina spinal fusions. The lamina becomes enormously thickened (Fig. 10.9) and causes symmetrical constriction of the vertebral canal from behind. On standard radiographic studies and myelography, the nature of this posterior compression will not be discernible. On other occasions, stenosis symptoms follow instability at the narrow segment proximal to the fusion.

3. Permits measurement

The assessment of the significance of various measurements of the spine is in its infancy and the long term practical clinical application of this CT facility is not known. The scanner permits an accurate measurement of the degree of rotation of the vertebra in conditions such as idiopathic scoliosis

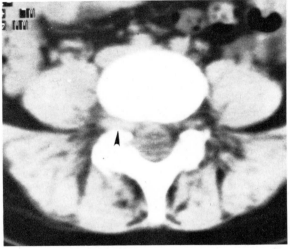

B

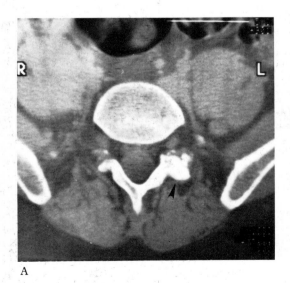

A

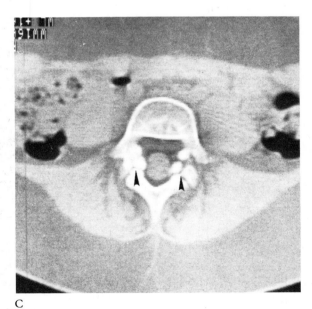

C

Fig. 10.8 (a, b, c) The 'rattle' of a spondylolisthesis due to cartilage and/or bone overgrowth is clearly shown by CT scanning (a). Perhaps it gained its name from its resemblance to a baby's rattle. Soft tissue (b) and bone (c) can be demonstrated encroaching into the root canal.

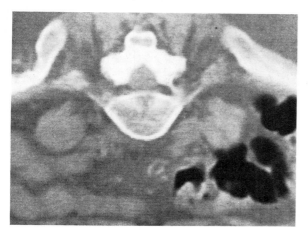

Fig. 10.9 Spinal stenosis due to thickening of the lamina following previous interlaminar fusion was an entity not radiologically demonstrable until the advent of CT scanning.

(Fig. 10.10): measurement of the inclination of a vertically orientated plane such as the angle of the facet joints (Fig. 10.11A): and precise physical measurements in the transverse plane for spinal stenosis (Fig. 10.11B,C,D). It is important to remember that because one has the ability to make a measurement accurately, it does not mean that the measurement has clinical significance. Many narrow canals are symptomless.

4. Assists invasive procedures

The precise depth of a lesion to be biopsied can be measured from the skin surface and furthermore the scanner does permit one to be sure of the accuracy of biopsy (Fig. 10.12). It is the only method of guiding the needle to a lesion which is demonstrable only by CT scanning.

TISSUE DIFFERENTIATION

CT scanning can measure, identify and therefore record, 2000 different radiation absorptions between air (black) and lead (white) and can differentiate tissues whose radiation absorptions are similar but

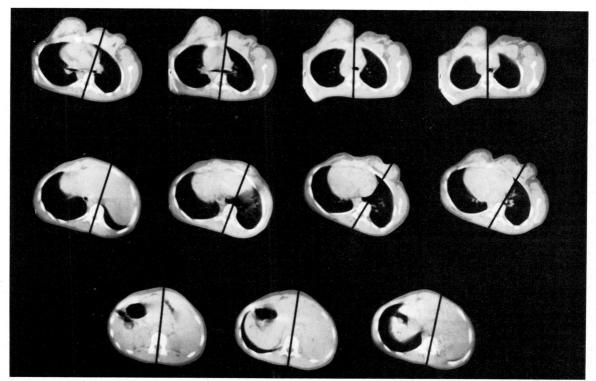

Fig. 10.10 A composite CT scan demonstrates the ease with which rotation of any particular spinal segment can be compared to any other segment. The accuracy of the measurement of vertebral rotation by CT scanning does not vary with the amount of rotation as it does with other techniques.

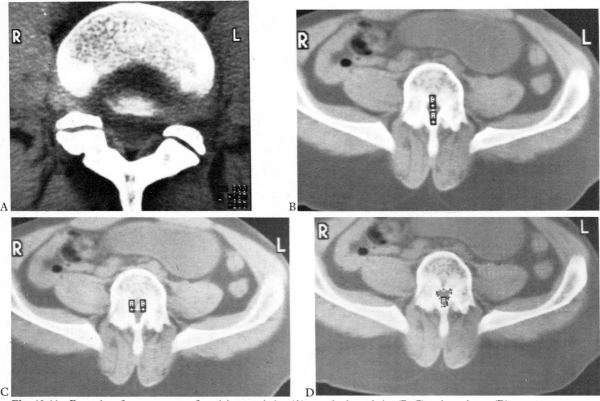

Fig. 10.11   Examples of measurements: facet joint angulation (A), vertebral canal size (B, C) and canal area (D).

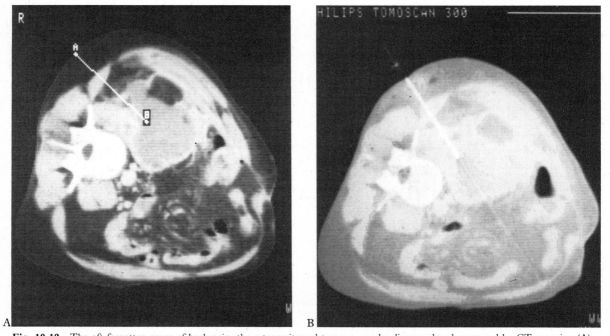

Fig. 10.12   The oft forgotten cause of back pain, the retroperitoneal tumour, can be diagnosed and measured by CT scanning (A) and biopsied under CT control (B). (Published with kind permission of Dr H Irving, St James's University Hospital).

not identical. This tissue differentiation is on a basis of radiation absorption and not on histological characteristics. Tissues which are entirely different histologically may undergo pathological processes which make their radiation absorptions similar and their differentiations will become impossible. Some tissues which are histologically totally dissimilar may have identical radiation absorptions and this too will prevent their differentiation. Finally, the CT scanner cannot reliably differentiate fluid from solid. If these failings are not understood, false negative CT scans can occur. Tissue differentiation is a valid concept whereas tissue diagnosis is not.

1. Permits a specific diagnosis

Intraspinal lipoma frequently accompanies dysraphism and needs to be excluded by CT scanning before surgical correction. Because fat is so much more radiolucent than any other tissue, the presence of a lipoma can be confidently diagnosed in the presence of a radiolucent tumour. We should remember the significance of mid line lipomas and attempt to show an intraspinal component (Fig. 10.13). It is not correct to assume that a fat containing tumour is benign and the word 'lipoma' is used to embrace all fatty tumours rather than just the benign.

The enhancement of vascular tumours by injected contrast medium should allow a reliable diagnosis of spinal angioma but experience is limited. Although the diagnosis is possible, the examination will probably not provide information that is of practical therapeutic benefit.

Small quantities of extradural air have been

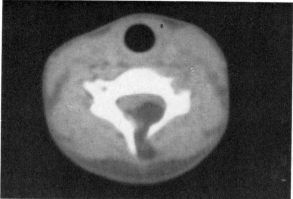

B

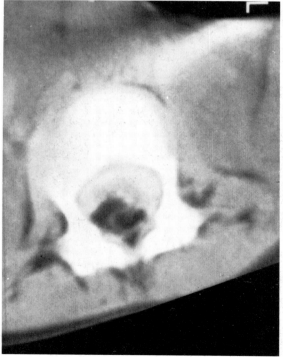

A

C

Fig. 10.13 The low attenuation of fat allows the lipoma of spinal dysraphism to be diagnosed with confidence. That a midline extraspinal lipoma (A) is significant is appreciated when the CT scan demonstrates an intraspinal component (B). Scanning can also demonstrate that a lipoma is infiltrating the nerve elements (C). (Published with kind permission of Dr J Lamb, St James's University Hospital).

accepted as diagnostic of a torn annulus when an intradiscal 'vacuum defect' communicates with the extra dural space. This sign of disc degeneration has no significance in the post operative spine.

2. To assess bone density

CT scanning of bone with x-rays of different potentials will allow calculation of the mineral content of that bone. This technique is still experimental but it should allow a precise assessment of bone mineral content and thereby identify osteoporosis, the replacement of bone by tumour, and expanded bone marrow, at a stage hitherto impossible.

3. Demonstrate disease recurrence

CT scanning may sometimes demonstrate recurrence of tumour. One can either use CSF as a contrast medium to demonstrate the presence of tumour within the dural sac or the encroachment of lesions on extradural fat (Fig. 10.14). The high incidence of false negative examinations from CT scanning does limit its value and one hesitates to propose its use in isolation.

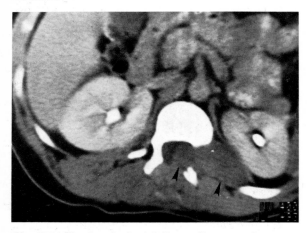

Fig. 10.14 The size of a dumb-bell neurofibroma can be assessed accurately pre-operatively or, as in this case, at the time of recurrence.

4. Demonstate extent of disease

The ability of the CT scanner to differentiate soft tissues does permit the reliable demonstration of the extent of extra spinal lesions. Retroperitoneal tumours are a cause of back pain which can be visualised by CT scan (Fig. 10.12).

The extension of spinal disease into the retroperitoneum or the paravertebral tissues can be precisely localised and assessed with scanning. An example of a neurofibroma at T 11 which has an extensive dumb-bell configuration with lateral growth as far as the left kidney is shown in Fig. 10.14. The presence and extent of spinal abscess (Fig. 10.15A,B) and spinal tumour (Fig. 10.15C) can also be demonstrated, and is particularly of value when planning surgical extirpation.

SPECIAL SITUATIONS

1. Trauma

Those of us who spend most of our time looking at standard radiographs tend to forget that oblique fractures aligned supero-inferiorly are invisible on frontal and lateral x-rays. Previously, it was felt that the appropriate oblique projection would demonstrate these otherwise invisible fractures, but the advent of CT scanning has shown just how astonishingly common are fractures which are not visible on any standard radiographic study. It is quite clear that one's entire concept of the significance of bone injury to the spine will have to be reconsidered in the light of this additional information.

Standard radiographs also tend to under-estimate the amount of bone that is displaced into the vertebral canal in such injuries as burst fracture. It is not at all unusual for the CT scan to show the vertebral canal filled with bone (Fig. 10.16) even though standard films may show little abnormality.

CT scanning has a vital role to play in deciding the management of the patient with a spinal cord injury.

2. Spinal stenosis

The supero-inferior projection of the spine is ideal for demonstrating anomalies in shape or size of the bony vertebral canal and, in addition, the soft tissue encroachment on the canal due to thickening of the ligamenta flava (Fig. 10.17) or of the lateral joint capsules. However, the CT scanner cannot show

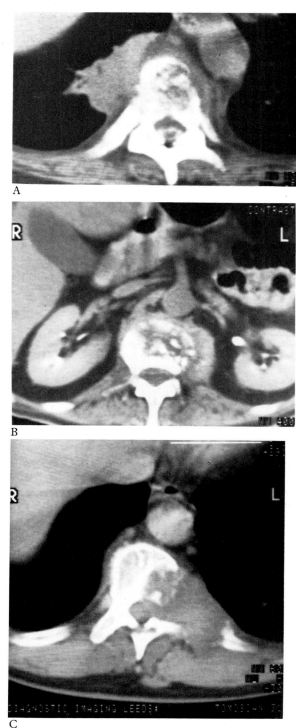

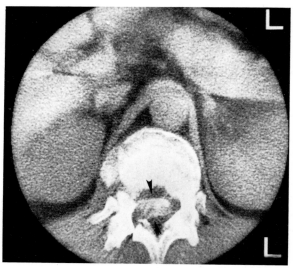

Fig. 10.16 The amount of bone herniated into the vertebral canal following injury is often much more than is suspected from standard radiographs. (Published with kind permission of Dr I Holland, St James's University Hospital).

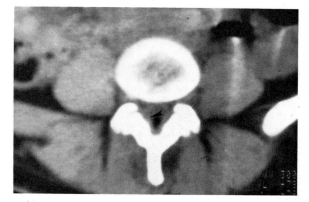

Fig. 10.17 Thickening of the ligamenta flava is a common finding of doubtful significance.

Fig. 10.15 It may be possible to differentiate between vertebral osteomyelitis (A,B) and metastatic tumour (C) but one would hesitate at present to rely on CT scanning exclusively.

significant spinal encroachment in patients whose myelogram is normal. If the vertebral canal is encroached by thickening of the bones and/or soft tissues, the narrowing will be apparent on a contrast study because the dural volume is decreased while the volume of nerve root is not and the proportion of contrast medium to nerve root will alter (Fig. 10.18), allowing one to diagnose a reduction in vertebral canal volume. Because the reduction is obliquely postero-lateral in origin in spinal stenosis the actual cause of the narrowing may not be clearly demonstrable on myelography (Fig. 10.19). CT scanning is, therefore, valuable in demonstrating the

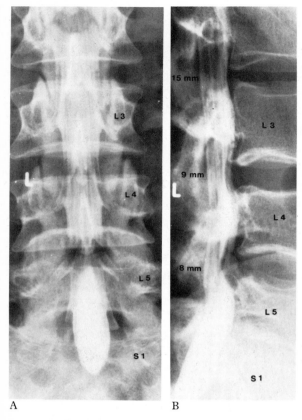

A   B

Fig. 10.18 The reduction of the volume of the vertebral canal in spinal stenosis can be appreciated from the myelogram. The proportion of nerve roots to contrast medium increases with the appearance of a canal crowded with nerve roots.

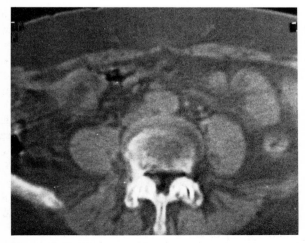

Fig. 10.19 Trefoil stenosed vertebral canal with adequate mid sagittal diameter.

precise nature of the cause of the stenosis rather than that a stenosis exists.

Those patients who have such severe narrowing of the vertebral canal that myelography is impossible, for example achondroplastic dwarfs, can be assessed only by CT scanning. Achondroplastics who develop paraplegia may have a significant stenosis also at the foramen magnum as well as the lumbar spine (Fig. 10.20). This may occur even in the presence of an adequate thoracic spinal canal (Lamb, 1983).

One must sometimes express caution to the diagnosis of 'spinal stenosis'. Many patients are mismanaged because of the presence of radiological features of 'spinal stenosis' in the presence of a clinical picture of single level disease. In such patients, a narrow or shallow vertebral canal should not be considered an indication for treatment but at the most only a hint of the aetiology and/or the prognosis. Patients who have spinal stenosis are indeed, more seriously disabled by single level disc disease but that must not mean that treatment of all the stenotic levels is required.

There are occasions, of course, when multiple level stenosis is clinically significant, and requires decompression. The CT scanning demonstration of antero-posterior diameters below 1.5 cms has tended to confirm the previous work by Porter and others who suggested that patients with symptomatic disc lesions tended to have small vertebral canals. It does not mean that the canal needs radical treatment. Antero-posterior measurements of the vertebral canal between 1.0 and 1.5 cms are a routine observation in patients who are having CT scanning for back pain and it is such a common finding that unless there is a compromising lesion no specific significance can be attached to it in the individual patient.

Neither does the presence of localised spinal stenosis either in the lateral recesses or in the root canal indicate the presence of symptoms or the need for treatment. Limited space may increase risk, but we must be cautious in interpreting an anatomical abnormality as responsible for a clinical picture.

3. The acute disc protrusion

Any assessment of the place of CT scanning in the patient with symptomatic disc protrusion must take into consideration the following two points. Firstly, patients with herniated intervertebral discs may have

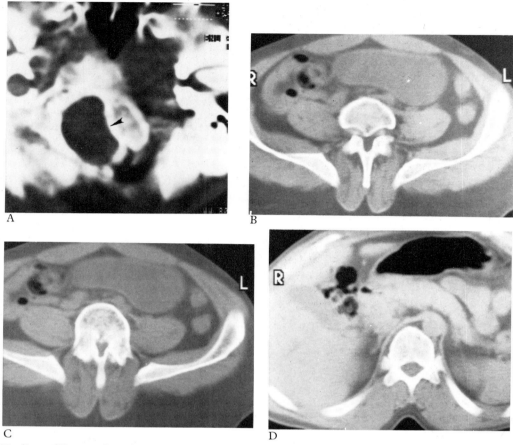

Fig. 10.20 Shows CT scans of an achondroplastic patient with stenosis of the foramen magnum (A) lumbar stenosis (B, C) but an adequate thoracic canal (D). (Published with kind permission of Dr J Lamb, St James's University Hospital).

a normal myelogram and a positive CT scan (Fig. 10.21) and secondly, they may have an abnormal myelogram and a negative CT scan (Fig. 10.22). Although the latter situation is more common with huge disc hernias it also occurs with the small hernia. It is possible to demonstrate a disc hernia if it encroaches on the extradural fat or where it is of different radiation absorption from the surrounding contents, but it is impossible to exclude a disc hernia in a situation where there is no demonstrable extradural fat (Fig. 10.22) or where pathological processes have so altered the radiation absorption of the dura that there is no difference between the herniated material and the dural contents (usually a massive disc hernia).

Useful diagnostic investigations can be divided into those with a very low false negative rate which are useful for screening, and those with a very low false positive rate which are useful for directing management. Examinations which have a significant number of both false positive and false negative results are not useful. CT scanning fits into the category of an examination with very few false positive results in which an anatomical abnormality on CT will usually be present at surgery, and this can be used to direct management. It does not mean, of course, that because a lesion is demonstrated, it is responsible for symptoms. By contrast, a negative CT examination does not exclude significant pathology. It is reasonable, therefore, to use CT scanning as the initial special diagnostic test on the patient suspected of having disc herniation and if the examination is positive, definitive treatment can begin. If the examination is not positive, myelography should be

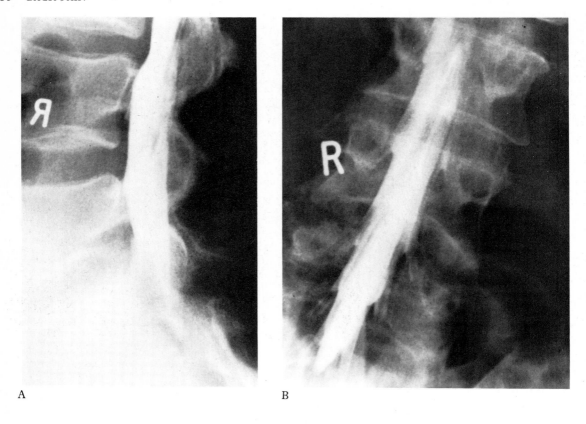

A   B

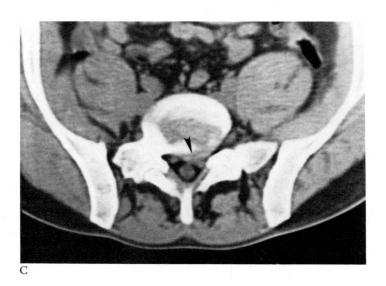

C

Fig. 10.21 A 'normal' myelogram and a positive CT scan in disc herniation.

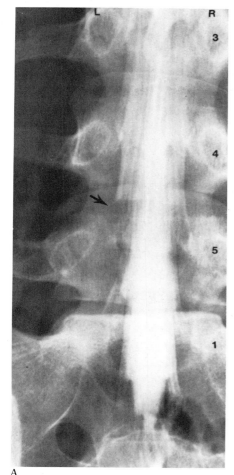

A

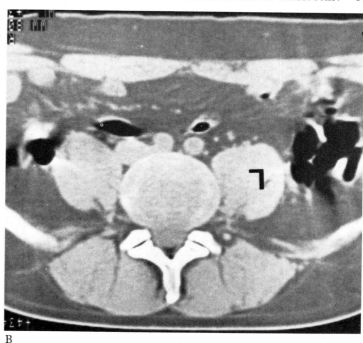

B

Fig. 10.22 A positive myelogram and a negative CT scan in disc herniation.

performed; a negative CT examination must be ignored. If this approach is followed, the majority of patients will be spared a myelogram but the false negative CT scan will be corrected by myelogram.

CT scanning is not a useful tool for examining large areas and it is, therefore, of limited value in excluding anatomical abnormalities that might give rise to a neurological deficit. Because of this, and because of its significant false negative rate, its use without myelography cannot be supported in patients who have a true neurological deficit.

There has been an unfortunate tendency to consider CT scanning an adversary of myelography rather than a companion, and discussions of CT scanning versus myelography tend to obscure the much more important place of CT scanning as an aid in helping with the understanding of abnormalities demonstrated by myelography.

4. Post laminectomy

The purpose of the radiological investigation of the symptomatic post laminectomy back is the same purpose of the radiological investigation of the unoperated back, namely to demonstrate the location of a surgically correctable lesion. As yet, there is no reliable method of differentiating by CT scanning herniated disc tissue from extradural scar tissue. It is reasonable to attempt to demonstrate a localised extra dural mass (Fig. 10.23) be it scar tissue or reherniated disc since both are treatable surgically. Even if it were possible to demonstrate a small localised reherniation in the midst of a mass of extradural scar tissue one must question the practical value of such a diagnosis.

Even though the return is so small, because the post laminectomy back can be such a problem there is a reasonable argument for routine use of CT scanning

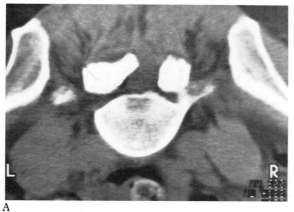

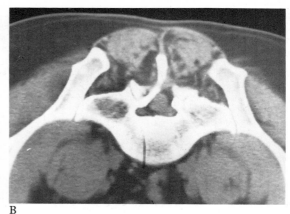

A   B

Fig. 10.23   The approach to the post-operative back should be to search for a localised extradural mass (A) rather than to attempt to differentiate reherniation from scan tissue. It is difficult to believe that a fragment of herniated disc in the middle of widespread post-operative scarring (B) could be significant.

along with myelography in the assessment of the post laminectomy patients.

5. To confirm normal

Intact extradural fat (Fig. 10.24) conclusively excludes encroachment on the vertebral canal. Similarly, other fat or air containing structures can be used to exclude the presence of disease encroaching on other areas. In this circumstance, the diagnosis of normal is possible. In all other circumstances, the failure to demonstrate the presence of disease by CT scanning does not indicate the absence of disease but only that it had not been demonstrated. We have false comfort if we interpret negative as normal.

In summary, CT scanning is first most valuable for the patient with back pain as a tool to answer questions posed by other forms of investigation. It is occasionally of value in making a precise anatomical diagnosis. On rare occasions it is able to make a precise pathological diagnosis and infrequently it will exclude disease. On no occasion can it demonstrate 'pain'.

Fig. 10.24 The demonstration of normal extradural fat excludes encroachment on the vertebral canal and in this situation the diagnosis of 'normal' (i.e. the absence of disease) is possible. If extradural fat is not visible (Fig. 10.22) disease cannot be excluded and the diagnosis is 'negative' (i.e. disease has not been shown).

REFERENCES

Dorwart R H and Genant H K 1983. Anatomy of the lumbar spine. The Radiological Clinics of North America 21: No 2 201–220

Haughton V M 1983. Computed tomography of the spine. Churchill Livingstone, London.
Lamb J 1983. Personal communication.
Robinson P J 1983. Use and abuse of whole body computed tomography. Up-date 853–867.

11

The place of diagnostic ultrasound in back pain management

We introduced ultrasound in 1978 as a method of measuring the oblique sagittal diameter of the vertebral canal, and have examined many thousands of patients and volunteer subjects. The technique does produce an impressive two dimensional display of echoes — the B-scan (Fig. 11.1) demonstrating vertebral body and laminar echoes. The distance between the reflecting surfaces of these echoes can be measured from the B-scan with electronic calipers (Asztely, 1983) or more precisely from an A-scan display at any one particular level (Fig. 11.2). There has been much debate about the accuracy, repeatability and relevance of the measurements.

ACCURACY

It has been suggested that it is not technically possible to use ultrasound to measure to an accuracy of less than half a wave-length. Using a 1.5 Mhz transducer, half a wave-length is 0.5 mm, and this is the range resolution. It is not possible to differentiate two surfaces closer together than this. The accuracy of the technique is therefore said to be questionable when measuring to a decimal place of a millimeter. The limitations of range resolution however, does not mean that. It does not mean that the measurement between two widely separated surfaces is also limited

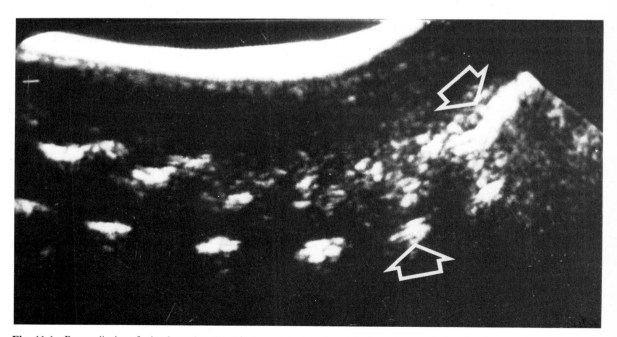

Fig. 11.1 B-scan display of a lumbar spine showing the vertebral body and lamina echoes, and the 'silent' vertebral canal. Arrows indicate echoes from the fifth lumbar vertebral body and echoes from the sacral laminae.

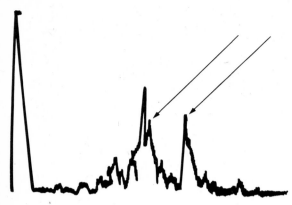

Fig. 11.2 A-scan display indicating the echoes believed to be reflected from the boundaries of the vertebral canal, the first arrow from the cranial lip of the dura, and the second from the posterior surface of the vertebral body.

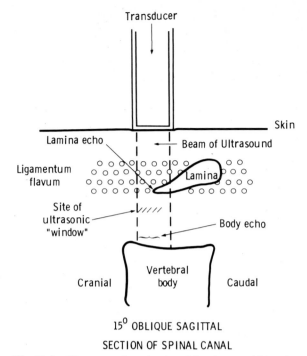

Fig. 11.3 Diagram to show the site of the ultrasound beam in the 15 degree oblique sagittal plane and the probable origin of the echoes.

by the range resolution. In practice, the accuracy of the diasonograph using a 1.5 Mhz transducer allows for detection of 0.05 mm movement of a reflecting surface fixed to a micrometer screw gauge. Such accuracy is highly acceptable for spinal measurement.

REPEATABILITY

Some have criticised the method on the grounds of poor repeatability (Stockdale and Finlay, 1980, Finlay et al, 1981) though with care and time we have been able to obtain a mean repeatability of less than 0.5 mm (Hibbert et al, 1981). It is true that many of the repeated measurements have a discrepancy of 0.5 mm, which is not inconsiderable when we are interested in a vertebral canal range from 11 to 18 mm. Legg (1982) thought the repeatability was adequate for epidemiological studies.

ANATOMICAL RELEVANCE

We confess we are unsure about the exact origin of the echoes. Our first and present impression is that they are from the cranial aspect of the posterior surface of the vertebral bodies and from the posterior margin of the canal at the cranial lip of the lamina (Fig. 11.3). Much of the sound must enter the canal through the ligamentum flavum. We are not convinced that we can identify echoes from soft tissues. On the other hand Aszteley (1983) and

Kadziolka et al (1981) conclude from cadaveric work that the echoes they measure originate from the boundaries between the dural sac and surrounding tissues at the level of the intervertebral disc. This may indeed be the echo from the posterior boundary, where the dura and the cranial lip of the lamina are closely opposed, but if the dura were the echo from the anterior boundary, we would have expected to recognise gross reduction of measurements with a large disc herniation. It would indeed be helpful to identify the site of the disc indenting the dura, but this is not our experience.

The fact that the ultrasound beam is of large area and must inevitably average to a point measurement, adds a further question to what point is actually being measured; the beam width will also vary with the focus of the transducer.

CLINICAL RELEVANCE

Some agree that measurement is possible, with a fair degree of repeatability, but that it has little clinical significance. Howie et al (1983) discard the technique because the pre-operative measurements bear no relationship with the observed level of pathological problem found at surgery. If indeed bony parameters are being measured, it is unlikely that ultrasound will show the clinical level of significant pathology, which is more often a combination of bone and soft tissue encroachment. They noted, but failed to comment upon, the fact that half their operated patients had vertebral canals in the bottom ten per cent of their 'normal values' from healthy volunteers.

We have found ultrasound measurements to be meaningful in certain clinical situations, and the results of population studies to be interesting epidemiologically. The general uncertainties of ultrasound however, has meant that the criticisms are widely accepted and it is not a diagnostic aid that has received general acceptance.

APPLICATION

The attraction of ultrasound as a diagnostic tool lies in its simplicity and safety for the patient (Figs. 11.4, 11.5). We routinely scan every back pain patient, and recognising the margin of error in the results, we are usually able to comment on the significance of space in the vertebral canal when talking to the patient at the end of the consultation. It is possible to explain to the patient with recurrent episodes of back pain, who frequently finds himself listing to one side, and yet has never had sciatic pain, that though he may have a disc producing back pain, he is fortunate to have an adequate vertebral canal protecting the nerve root.

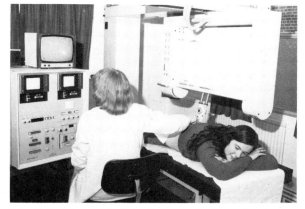

Fig. 11.4 Photograph of the diasonograph. The patient lies prone and the gantry is fixed at 15 degrees to the sagittal plane.

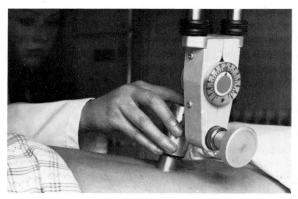

Fig. 11.5 The transducer is moved along the lumbar spine, a few centimetres lateral to the spinous processes.

For the next young patient with leg pain and poor straight leg raising, the narrow canal is discussed as a persisting vulnerability, with need for a great deal of respect.

A narrow canal with an unstable segment makes talk about dural pain sensible. So many patients with rising expectations about health, want to know as much as possible about the source of pain, and ultrasound does give that opportunity to answer some of their questions in a logical manner.

Neurogenic claudication

Neurogenic claudication is associated with a shallow vertebral canal, just one factor in the pathogenesis of the condition, but an essential factor. If the possibility of surgery is contemplated, myelography or a CT scan is essential, but there are some patients not sufficiently disabled for surgery, or with inappropriate signs, where one would withhold invasive investigations. An ultrasound scan in the upper percentiles would suggest a diagnosis other than neurogenic claudication.

Isthmic spondylolisthesis

Forward displacement of the proximal vertebral body is usually obvious from the ultrasound echoes (Fig. 11.6), and at the level of displacement the canal measurements are generally wider than in other patients. This may be because the displaced lamina increases the sagittal diameter, or because the canal is usually dome-shaped and rarely trefoil in spondylolisthesis, or because about a third of the patients have a coexistent spina bifida.

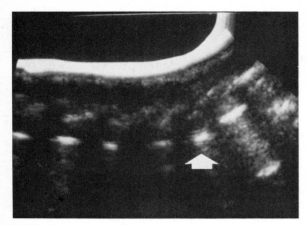

Fig. 11.6 B-scan display of patient with isthmic spondylolisthesis at L.5/S.1 showing forward displacement of the L.5 body echo.

Intra-operative ultrasonography

Eismont et al (1984) have found real time ultrasonography a useful adjunct in spinal surgery allowing better definition of spinal tumours, anterior bony encroachment from trauma, stenosis and disc herniation. Endoscopic ultrasonography is a new development.

Epidemiologically our ultrasound results suggest that the depth of the vertebral canal is an important factor in most patients with back pain. In a general practice study (Drinkall et al, 1984) we found that patients attending with back pain had significantly smaller measurements than a randomised group of matched controls without any previous attendance with back pain. Patients attending hospital with back pain, when compared with volunteers of similar age, tended to have narrower canals, 39 per cent of clinic patients being below the tenth percentile of the volunteers, 43 per cent of those admitted, and 46 per cent of those having spinal surgery being below the tenth percentile (Fig. 11.7).

Forsberg and Walloe (1982) reported that B-scan measurements for their patients who had made a poor recovery from disc surgery, were narrower than for those who had recovered uneventfully.

An industrial study showed that 37 per cent of the days lost from work by a group of coal miners over 50 years of age was by the ten per cent of men with

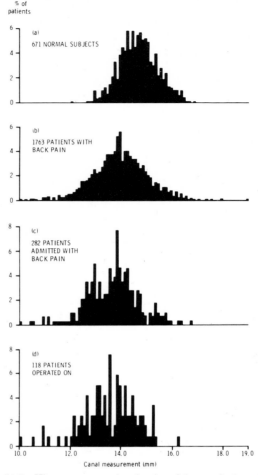

Fig. 11.7 Histogram comparing the size of the vertebral canal at L.5 in age matched asymptomatic subjects, patients attending hospital with low back pain, patients admitted with low back pain, and those requiring spinal surgery.

narowest canals (Macdonald et al, 1984) (Fig. 11.8). In the three years after measurement, the men who took early retirement had significantly narrower canals than those who stayed at work. It seems that the canal size as measured by ultrasound, has some value in predicting those most vulnerable to back pain. The implications for occupational health are considerable.

Population studies using ultrasound in three distinct back pain syndromes, throws some light on their pathogenesis. 41 per cent of our patients with symptomatic disc lesions had canal measurements below the tenth percentile for asymptomatic volunteers (Table 1) suggesting that for many, the

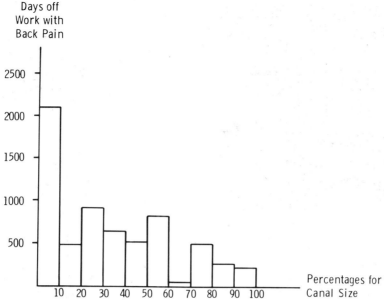

Fig. 11.8 Histogram of days lost from work due to back pain by miners over 50 years of age, according to canal size. 32 per cent of days lost from work was by men below the 10th percentile.

Table 11.1 Comparison of ultrasound canal measurements in patients with symptomatic disc lesion, root entrapment syndrome and neurogenic claudication

Clincal diagnosis	Number of patienta	% male	Age (years)	Mean canal measurements (cms)	Age range of controls	Mean canal measurements (cms)	5th	10th	50th
					Comparison with volunteer subjects		% of patients below percentile		
Disc lesion	173	71.8	33.6± 6.6	L.1 1.53±0.13	20–50	1.54±0.08	36.4	41.0	82.7
				L.2 1.49±0.13	(n–547)	1.52±0.08			
				L.3 1.43±0.12		1.49±0.07			
				L.4 1.38±0.11		1.46±0.08			
				L.5 1.38±0.12		1.48±0.08			
Neurogenic claudication	134	70.1	50.8±10.7	1.48±0.11	40–60	1.54±0.07	42.5	56.7	85.1
				1.44±0.11	(n–197)	1.51±0.08			
				1.38±0.10		1.47±0.08			
				1.33±0.10		1.45±0.08			
				1.33±0.12		1.46±0.08			
Root entrapment syndrome	250	52.7	51.3± 7.8	1.51±0.10	40–60	1.54±0.07	21.2	30.0	67.2
				1.48±0.10	(n–197)	1.51±0.08			
				1.43±0.09		1.47±0.08			
				1.49±0.10		1.45±0.08			
				1.41±0.10		1.46±0.08			

canal size is an important factor in the pain mechanism. This is more significant in our older patients whose back pain restricts walking distance; 57 per cent were below the tenth percentile. In root entrapment syndrome, where the lesion is more lateral in the root canal, only 30 per cent had central canal measurements below the tenth percentile.

In back pain syndromes associated with vertebral displacement, the canal size as measured by ultrasound seems to have variable significance. It assumes greater importance when pain is associated with retrololisthesis or rotationary displacement (43 per cent below the tenth percentile), some importance in degenerative spondylolisthesis, and less in isthmic spondylolisthesis (Table 2).

Ultrasound has its limitations, even if one accepts a fair degree of accuracy, repeatability and anatomical relevance. It has not been shown to help in the prediction of outcome of an episode of back pain, in the likelihood of a recurrence within 12 months (Drinkall et al, 1984), nor will it make the diagnosis of the level of significant pathology. It does make us think about space in the vertebral canal, however, and if we understand its limitations, it may yet prove to be a useful tool.

There is no question at all that space within the vertebral canal is of great clinical significance. An individual with a shallow canal and especially a trefoil shaped canal at L.5, has a highly vulnerable back, and is a subject at risk. The question still to be answered is whether this individual can reliably be identified by ultrasound.

Table 11.2 Comparison of ultrasound canal measurements in patients with vertebral displacement

	Number of patients	% male	Age (years)	Mean canal measurements (cms)	Comparison with volunteer subjects		% of patients below percentile		
					Age range of controls	Mean canal measurements (cms)	5th	10th	50th
Retro-spondylolisthesis	56	62.1	45.5±12.4	1.48±0.09	30–60	1.54±0.07	21.4	42.9	89.3
				1.45±0.09	(n–557)	1.51±0.07			
				1.41±0.08		1.48±0.08			
				1.38±0.08		1.45±0.08			
				1.39±0.06		1.47±0.08			
Degenerative spondylolisthesis	65	28.4	61.3±10.3	1.48±0.09	50–65	1.54±0.08	23.1	32.3	78.5
				1.45±0.09	(n–124)	1.51±0.08			
				1.42±0.08		1.47±0.09			
				1.39±0.09		1.45±0.08			
				1.39±0.10		1.47±0.08			
Isthmic spondylolisthesis	89	64.4	39.3±13.5	1.52±0.09	30–50	1.54±0.07	16.9	24.7	67.4
				1.49±0.09	(n–315)	1.52±0.07			
				1.46±0.07		1.49±0.07			
				1.44±0.09		1.46±0.08			
				1.43±0.11		1.47±0.07			

REFERENCES

Asztely M 1983 Lumbar sonography: a comparative radiological study. Thesis: Departments of diagnostic radiology and orthopaedic surgery, University of Goteborg, Sweden

Drinkall J N, Porter R W, Hibbert C S, Evans C 1984 The value of ultrasonic measurement of the spinal canal diameter in general practice. British Medical Journal 288: 121–122

Eismont F, Morse B, Post J D, Brown M, Rauschning W, Green B and Quencer R 1984 Intra-operative ultrasonogrphy of the lumbar spine presented to the International Society for Study of the Lumbar Spine, Montreal

Finlay D, Stockdale H R, Lewin E 1981 An appraisal of the use of diagnostic ultrasound to quantify the lumbar spinal canal. British Journal of Radiology 54: 870–874

Forsbert L, Walloe A 1982 Ultrasound in sciatica. Acta orthop. Scand. 53: 393–395

Hibbert C S, Delaygue C, McGlen B, Porter R W 1981 Measurement of the lumbar spinal canal by diagnostic ultrasound. British Journal of Radiology 54: 905–907

Howie D W, Chatterron B E, Hone M R 1983 Failure of ultrasound in the investigation of sciatica. Journal of Bone and Joint Surgery 65–B: 144–147

Kadziolka R, Asztely M, Hanai K, Hansson T, Nachemson A 1981 Ultrasonic measurement of the lumbar spinal canal. Journal of Bone and Joint Surgery 63–B: 504–507

Legg S J, Gibbs V 1982 Measurement of the lumbar spinal canal by echo ultrasound. Spine

Macdonald E B, Porter R, Hibbert C, Hart J 1984 The relationship between spinal canal diameter and back pain in coal miners: ultrasonic measurement a screening test? Journal of Occupational Medicine 26: 23–28

Porter R W, Wicks M, Ottewell D 1978 Measurement of the spinal canal by diagnostic ultrasound. Journal of Bone and Joint Surgery 60–B, No. 4, 481–485

Stockdale H R, Finlay D 1980 Use of diagnostic ultrasound to measure the lumbar spinal canal. British Journal of Radiology 53: 1101–1102

12

Herniated nucleus pulposus — pathology, diagnosis and management

PATHOLOGY

Mixter and Barr (1934) first described the clinical significance of disc herniation and the results of surgical excision. The diagnosis became so fashionable that almost all backache was attributed to the intervertebral disc. Perhaps it has now taken its rightful place as a common source of acute and chronic disability, but even when responsible for symptoms, it is one factor amongst many.

Disruption of the inner fibres of the posterior annulus will cause the nucleus to bulge, especially when loaded, and result in a space-occupying protrusion into the anterior aspect of the vertebral canal. If the more peripheral fibres of the annulus are also torn or separated, the protrusion will increase in size, and finally rupture through the outer fibres as a nuclear hernia. A disc is extruded when the displaced nuclear material within the vertebral canal is still connected to material within the disc (Fig. 12.1). It is sequestrated when nuclear material escapes into the vertebral canal as one or more free fragments (Fig. 12.2). The posterior longitudinal ligament and the fascial extension laterally generally prevents the disc material from rupturing freely into the canal, but this can occur, and free fragments migrate to other locations. A central protrusion is more effectively resisted by the strong posterior longitudinal ligament than a more lateral lesion. There can thus be considerable variation in both the site and the size of the lesion.

The speed of disc protrusion is yet another variable factor. A disc may bulge after disruption of the inner annular fibres, partially resolve to increase at a later time, and then eventually extrude years later. Alternatively, in a matter of hours, the nucleus of a second disc may rupture through the annulus, with no opportunity for repair to influence the outcome.

The disc lesion itself is very variable in its speed of

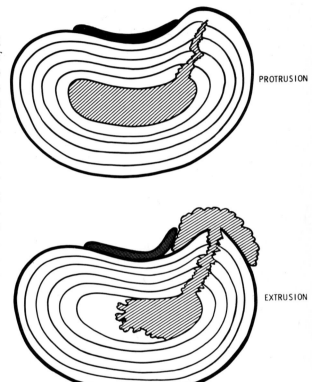

PROTRUSION

EXTRUSION

Fig. 12.1 Diagram to show an annular fissure allowing protrusion of the nucleus pulposis lateral to the posterior longitudinal ligament, and extrusion of the nucleus if the annular tear is complete.

development, its size and its site, but there are other factors than the disc which influence the symptomatology. If the lesion is important, the space which it occupies is highly relevant. This has for long been a neglected factor but we now know that a disc prolapse into a restricted space is more likely to produce troublesome symptoms than protrusion into a wider canal (Epstein et al, 1962, Porter et al, 1978).

Ultrasound measurements of the oblique sagittal

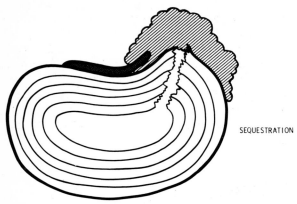

Fig. 12.2 The nucleus may herniate through the annular tear as a sequestration.

accommodate a disc protrusion without even dural pain. Root pain may be only first experienced later in life as a result of the degenerative changes in the root canal, the original disc having protruded symptomlessly in early adult life. The anomaly of disc disruption without symptoms is not surprising if one considers the variable size of the vertebral canal.

The shape of the canal is as important as the size, in the symptomatology of disc protrusion. A small dome-shaped canal may be troublesome, but a small trefoil shaped canal disastrous (Fig. 12.4). A trefoil configuration of a large canal may not be such a problem, depending on how far laterally the disc bulge extends. A lesion far lateral into the root canal

diameter of the vertebral canal in patients with root symptoms and signs from acute disc pathology, show that nearly half of them have canal measurements in the bottom ten per cent of the population (Fig. 12.3). It is reasonable to assume that subjects with wider canals are equally vulnerable to develop disc pathology, but that many do not experience root symptoms because there is sufficient space within the vertebral canal for the roots to avoid involvement. A protrusion into such a canal can cause dural irritation (Cyriax, 1978) with back pain, restricted movement and protective muscle spasm, but no root problems. A wide canal with adequate extra dural space, could

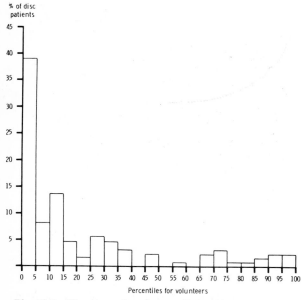

Fig. 12.3 Histogram of canal size at L.5 measured by ultrasound for patients with symptomatic disc lesions, compared with the percentile measurements of age matched volunteers.

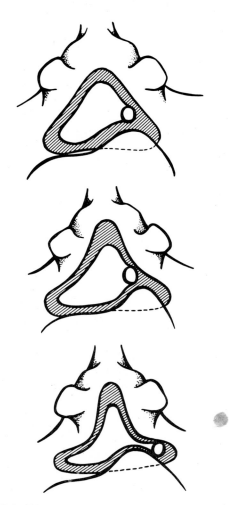

Fig. 12.4 Diagram to show that a nerve root may be spared from a protrusion into a dome shaped canal, is partly compromised from the same protrusion in a bell shaped canal, but is readily involved in a trefoil shaped canal.

will quickly involve the root irrespective of the canal's size and shape (Fig. 12.5).

Nerve roots tethered by dural ligaments (Spencer et al, 1983) and anomalous roots (Kadish and Simmons, 1984) will be more readily affected by disc protrusion, than freely mobile roots.

Disc encroachment through the posterior longitudinal ligament into the vertebral canal affects first the dura, and then the roots or ganglia of the cauda equina. We do not know how these structures produce pain, nor the relative importance of mechanical irritation, biochemical and ischaemic factors.

DIAGNOSIS

Symptomatic disc lesions occur more commonly in the male, and generally present in the fourth decade (Sprangfort, 1972) (Fig. 12.6). The manner of presentation is as diverse as the factors responsible. Sometimes we can be sure of the diagnosis, sometimes only suspicious.

PROBABLE LOWER LUMBAR DISC LESION

Pain in the lower back is usually the first symptom, but the diagnosis is made by root symptoms and

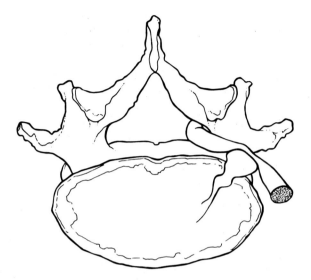

Fig. 12.5 Diagram to show involvement of an L.5 root in the root canal, from a central disc lesion, irrespective of the size of the central canal.

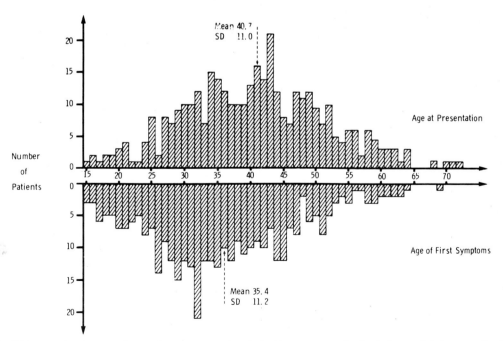

Fig. 12.6 Histogram showing age when patients present to hospital with a symptomatic disc lesion, and their age at the time of the first symptoms.

signs. Pain spreads or is replaced by pain first in the buttock, thigh, posterior calf and ankle. In an L.5 lesion, there may be pain or numbness in the big toe and with an S.1 lesion in the outer foot. It is generally worse with coughing, sneezing, laughing or straining. Its intensity is variable. In the younger patients, the symptoms are less marked than the signs. Many a young man will keep at work with a large lumbar disc lesion, with few symptoms other than stiffness of the back and legs.

An interesting phenomenon that accompanies a disc protrusion in about one third of the patients is a gravity induced list. The pelvis remains horizontal with the floor, but the lumbar spine deviates to one side with a 'wind-swept' appearance (Fig. 12.7). The list is abolished by lying down (Fig. 8.1, page 50), and by hanging on a bar (Fig. 12.8). It is not known if it

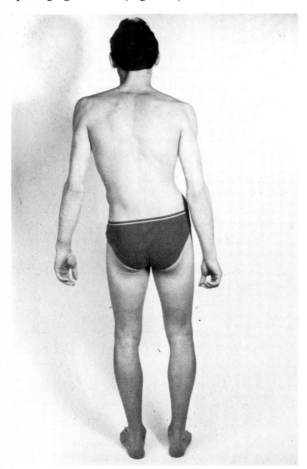

Fig. 12.7 The 'wind swept' appearance of a patient with a lower lumbar disc lesion listing to the left.

serves a useful function, but it does shift the centre of gravity from the central plane, altering the weight distribution when standing. This can be shown clearly when asking a patient with a list to stand first on the ipsilateral leg, when the list remains. By standing on the contralateral side, presumably altering the centre of gravity now serves no useful function, and the list can be apparently voluntarily corrected (Fig. 12.9). However, a radiograph shows that the correction, though moving the centre of gravity to the mid line is only apparent (Fig. 12.10). The lumbar scoliosis remains. The reflex spasm can only be abolished by lying down.

The psoas is the muscle probably mainly responsible for the list (Grieve, 1983), but the spinal mechanism is not understood. The list is almost always associated with a disc protrusion (Scott, 1983). We observed such a list in 5.6 per cent of patients attending a back pain clinic. Of 100 listing patients, 71 had pain in a sciatic distribution below the knee, and 49 fulfilled McCulloch's criteria for a symptomatic lumbar disc lesion. 20 subsequently had surgical excision of the disc. It is interesting that no patient with a list had isthmic spondylolisthesis, when perhaps disc protrusion is less common, or the wide canal is significant.

It has previously been suggested that a list has functional value, easing the root away from a protruding disc (Bianco, 1968, Patzold et al, 1975, Scott, 1983) but in our series of 20 listing patients who required disc surgery, there was no consistent topographical relationship between the disc, the root and the side of the list. It has also been suggested that a list is less likely to occur with a disc lesion at L.5/S.1 because of the powerful restraint of the ilio-lumbar ligaments, but this was not our experience. In fact, 12 had excision of the L.5/S.1 disc, 6 excision of L.4/5 and 2 the L.3/4 disc.

The fact that almost twice as many patients list to the left (66 compared with 31 to the right) suggests that a dominant reflex may be responsible for the laterality and there is evidence to support this (Porter and Miller, 1984). A few patients can demonstrate an alternating list (Remak, 1881, Capener, 1933) (Fig. 8.1, page 50), listing first to one side and then to the other.

Lumbar flexion and extension is limited probably because of dural irritation and corresponds to the limitation of straight leg raising. Lateral flexion is

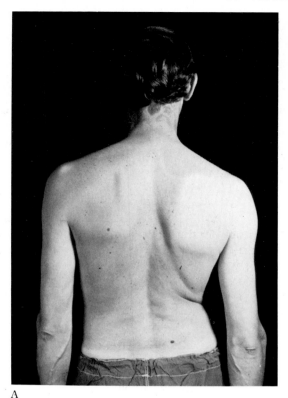

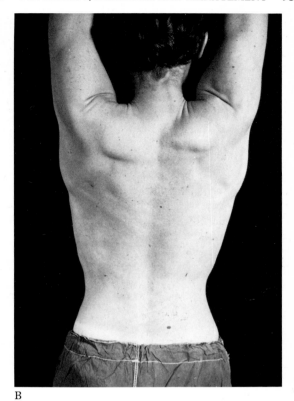

A   B

Fig. 12.8 a) The author, unable to correct a list, when standing.   b) The list is abolished by hanging from a bar.

unaffected. There is often a loss of normal lumbar lordosis.

Tenderness is well localised to the level of the disc lesion. Straight leg raising of 50 degrees or less is almost pathognomonic of a disc lesion, as is cross leg pain. Other tension tests reinforce these signs (page 54). The root responsible may be suggested from diminution of a knee or ankle reflex, motor weakness, wasting and sensory impairment but this does not necessarily help in identifying the offending disc. A disc lesion at L.4/5 level can cause L.4, L.5 or S.1 root symptoms, and a disc at L.5/S.1 can affect either the L.5 or S.1 root.

One can confidently make the diagnosis of a lumbar intervertebral disc lesion with such a history and collection of abnormal signs, even if it is not possible to identify the level, and if they persisted over a few weeks, it would be unusual to find a myelographic or CT examination normal.

McCulloch (1977) described several criteria which he thought should be present in order to make the diagnosis of a symptomatic disc lesion. He expected three of the following five criteria to be present:

1. Unilateral leg pain in a typical sciatic root distribution, including discomfort below the knee

2. Specific neurological symptoms incriminating a single nerve

3. Limitation of straight leg raising by at least 50 per cent of normal

4. At least two neurological changes of muscle wasting, muscle weakness, sensory change or hyporeflexia

5. Myelographic evidence of a disc protrusion.

PRESUMPTIVE LOWER LUMBAR DISC LESION

There are occasions when the diagnosis cannot be made with such confidence. The diagnosis is only presumptive, and yet symptoms and signs suggest a diagnosis of disc protrusion. Such a patient may have back pain associated with a gravity induced list, but

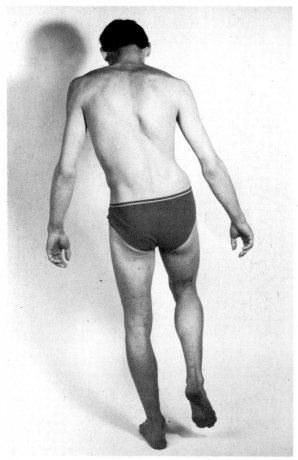

Fig. 12.9A Photograph of the patient in Fig. 7 now standing on the ipsilateral leg but the list cannot be corrected.

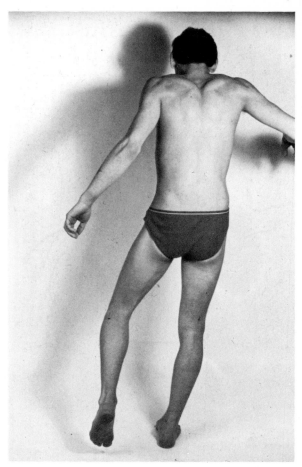

Fig. 12.9B Standing on the contra-lateral leg allows correction of the list.

no nerve root involvement, and no root signs; or there may be a minimal root lesion, with pain to the ankle, straight leg raising slightly reduced and no abnormal neurological signs. One would not over-investigate for the sake of a diagnosis, unless this was likely to affect management, and the diagnosis remains only speculative.

POSSIBLE LOWER LUMBAR DISC LESION

The natural history of a disc lesion which eventually requires surgical excision not infrequently begins with a mild episode of back pain and few abnormal signs. Gradually each episode may become worse until the full picture develops. We are justified,

therefore, in considering the possibility of a disc lesion with every acute attack of back pain, especially when there are occasional supporting signs. Any acute episode of back pain that limits spinal movement, that causes a list, reduces straight leg raising, that is aggravated by coughing, that puts a patient to bed, could be associated with a disc protrusion, that will one day declare itself.

MANAGEMENT

Conservative management

The best place to recover from a disc lesion is in bed. It has not been shown that anything is better. Some

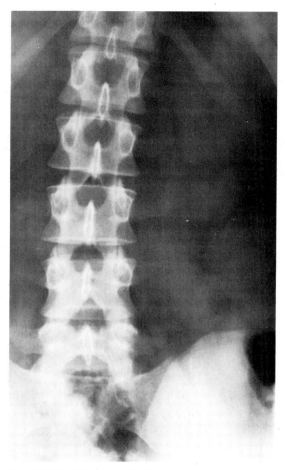

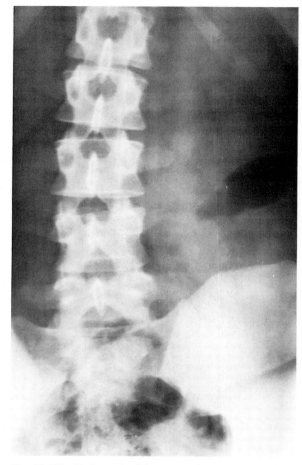

Fig. 12.10A AP radiograph of patient with symptomatic disc lesion listing to the left when standing. Centre of gravity is shifted to the left.

Fig. 12.10B Radiograph of the same patient standing on the right leg alone. The left pelvis is raised, the psoas contracted, and the centre of gravity is moved to the mid line. The scoliosis remains.

may work it off, others may be fortunate enough to have it manipulated away, but bed rest is the treatment of choice. To ignore the value of rest is to court trouble. Two weeks in bed is about right for most of the symptoms and signs to settle. A pillow under the knees can help, but the patient usually finds the most comfortable position for themselves. Food is taken in sandwich form, and a straw or a feeding cup prevents the spilling of fluids. Strict bed rest is important, except for toilet purposes. Initially analgesics may be needed around the clock, but they should be reduced as the pain settles, at least during the day. The back is never quite as good as it feels, and patients should be warned about taking short cuts

and leaving their bed too soon. Improved straight leg raising is a measure of progress. If it is still very limited after two weeks, in-patient bed rest should be considered.

It is difficult to account for the therapeutic effects of a hospital bed, but it is better than rest at home. Many an obdurate disc will settle with two weeks of in-patient care. Bed rest, letting the patient find their own position of comfort, or lying supine with the hips and knees flexed, is probably as good as traction. The common denominator for conservative in-patient treatment is an adequate period spent in the horizontal position.

If traction is applied, pelvic traction is preferable to

Pugh's leg traction when there is the possible complication of deep venous thrombosis. Pelvic traction also has its complications, with pain or numbness in the outer thigh from compression of the lateral cutaneous nerve. It calls for repositioning or removal of the corset. Lower abdominal pain, possibly from tension on the rectus muscles, is relieved by flexing the hips on a couple of pillows. No more than two pounds per stone body weight is necessary. It is applied gradually over a twelve hour period. The speed of application of the weights is dictated by any increase in discomfort. It may be necessary to stop for a period rather than have to reduce the weights later.

The best prognostic sign is straight leg raising, and it should return to almost 90 degrees before the patient is allowed home. One regrets allowing a patient home in less than two weeks, even if there appears to be a rapid recovery. It may take a third week of patience to obtain success.

Patients at this stage can be arbitrarily divided into three groups. The first are obviously better, with little discomfort, good straight leg raising, and no abnormal neurological signs. They can go home, stay off work a few weeks and expect a good result in the short term. They want to know how much exercise and how much rest is necessary, their future limitations, and how can recurrences be prevented. A 'Back School' programme is helpful at some time during the recovery phase (Chapter 23), ideally beginning in the recumbent period.

A second group are not better, but have made some progress. Straight leg raising may have increased from 20/70 to 60/80. Some abnormal neurological signs may have resolved, but perhaps sensory impairment remains. The experience of Weber (1983) is that these patients ultimately do as well treated conservatively as by operation. They can go home to have periods of rest, gradually increasing their activity over the weeks. Three months in a lightweight cast can help. Recovery may be slow, with further recurrences, but surgery does not offer a better prognosis. Chymonucleolysis experience is insufficient to predict the long term prognosis for this group of patients.

A third group fail to improve and require active treatment, either by surgically excising the disc, or by chymonucleolysis. If after three weeks in a hospital bed, straight leg raising is 50 degrees or less, it is worth identifying the disc by a radiculogram or CT scan, and treating it actively. Continuing cross leg pain and persistent motor weakness at this stage also predicts a probable failure of further conservative treatment.

One may be tempted to abandon conservative management if there is gross weakness of dorsiflexion of the foot or of the peronei. If however there is some motor improvement patience may be rewarded by full recovery. Discectomy becomes an emergency when bladder dysfunction follows a massive disc prolapse. A neurogenic bladder is the price for delay.

Surgery

Surgery is indicated for disc symptoms with bladder dysfunction and for disc symptoms with root pain that has failed to respond to conservative management. The decision to operate is not influenced by the radiculogram or CT scan, but demonstration of the site of the disc lesion does simplify the procedure (Fig. 12.11). The choice of investigation, radiculography or CT is dictated partly by the availability of the latter. Most comparative studies have shown similar overall accuracies for both techniques (Haughton et al, 1982, Fries et al, 1982), but Rothman et al (1984) found that metrizamide radiculography was superior to CT scan in specificity and sensitivity in the diagnosis of lumbar disc herniation. The difference was less apparent in the younger patient. In fact, CT may be slightly better at L.5/S.1 where physiological attenuation of the dural sac may present radiculographic problems (Williams et al, 1980). The usual CT signs are: material of soft tissue density extending from the posterior annulus into the vertebral canal; the protruded disc material having a greater density measurement than the adjacent theca; the epidural fat being obliterated at the site of the lesion; and indentation of the thecal sac or distortion of the nerve root (Teplick and Haskin, 1983).

The aim of disc surgery should be to remove the disc tissue that is producing pressure on the nerve root, with its resultant pain and neurological deficit, and to avoid immediate and late complications.

To achieve these aims, surgeons differ in their surgical preferences. Some choose a wide exposure (Paine and Haung, 1972, Shenkin and Hash, 1976, Choudhury and Taylor, 1976, Herron and Pheasant,

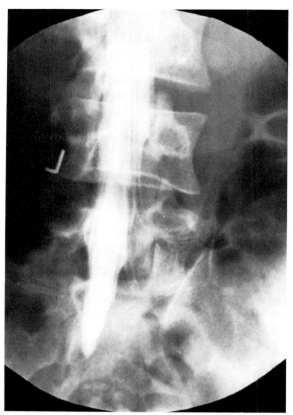

Fig. 12.11A Classical appearance of a disc lesion at L.5/S.1 with obliteration of the dural sheath of the left S.1 root.

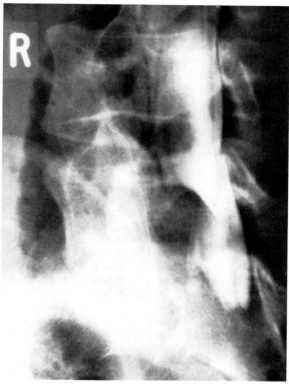

Fig. 12.11B A massive disc herniation at L.5/S.1 distorting the dural sac. Both discs (a) and (b) were easily removed through a small fenestration.

1983) and extensively remove bony structures. Some feel it is important to examine several discs, and follow the respective nerve roots visually. This minimises the risk of leaving behind sequestrated material that may have migrated, ensures that all the disc is removed from the canal, and that a second lesion is not neglected. If insufficient nuclear material is removed from within the annulus, there is a possibility of recurrence and if too much is removed, then disc space narrowing can produce late sequelae. Some add a spinal fusion to the discectomy though this appears to be of limited value (Frymoyer et al, 1978). Others advocate a small exposure and microdiscectomy (Williams, 1978, Hudgins, 1983) believing that it allows the surgeon to work more precisely, that it reduces complications and hastens recovery. A middle course is described here, removing the offending part of the disc through a fenestration.

The patient lies prone on an operating frame, with the abdomen dependant avoiding an increase in venous pressure. Semi flexion makes the operation easier by increasing the inter laminar space. An incision is made over the spinous processes of L.4, L.5 and S.1, and subcutaneous bleeding is minimised by keeping strictly to the mid line. Para spinal muscles are separated from the spinous processes and laminae, and the tendinous insertions of multifidus divided. Self retaining retractors provide both a good exposure and haemostasis. The fifth lumbar vertebra is identified by grasping the spinous processes with bone holders and noting the relative mobility of L.5 compared with S.1. Lumbarisation or sacralisation should not cause confusion if this has previously been identified radiographically. If the site of the disc lesion has been confidently identified by radiculography, and this corresponds with the clinical assessment, only one disc space need be exposed. A small window of the caudal aspect of the lamina above is removed with rongeurs and a square of ligamentum flavum excised. As the dura is gently displaced medially, a bulging disc is first felt with a dissector and then seen as a white protrusion. The displaced nerve root, responsible for the sciatica and tension signs, is identified and carefully retracted from the protrusion. It can be flattened like a ribbon over the disc material, and unless recognised, an apparent incision into the disc can cut the root or ganglion. It is important to consider the possibility of a conjoint root. It is an anomaly that occurs in at least 8 per cent of the population (Hasue et al, 1983, Kadish and Simmons, 1984) and makes the nerve root vulnerable to surgical injury. If the nucleus is extruded or sequestrated, it may be forced into the wound by the process of teasing away of the nerve root. The disc material can then be extracted in one piece (Fig. 12.12). A blunt dissector is inserted through the rent in the annulus into the nuclear space. Other

fragments of nucleus are removed with a disc extractor. When a disc is protruding, with some outer fibres of the annulus intact, it is necessary to make a cruciate incision in these fibres, and then extract the nuclear material. The limit of the nucleus is recognised by the feel of the tissue, but the remaining annulus should not be penetrated by the extractor. Generally, one or two large fragments are removed, and several smaller pieces.

At the end of the operation, the dura should be free and the nerve root mobile. If there is any doubt that some sequestrated material remains, further exposure is necessary, perhaps into the root canal, but provided the disc protrusion is unequivocal, there is no need to explore the other side or other levels. When the vertebral canal is particularly narrow, and trefoil in configuration, it is worth decompressing the central canal in addition to removing the prolapsed disc, and sometimes decompressing the root canal. There is no place for surgical exploration of the vertebral canal as

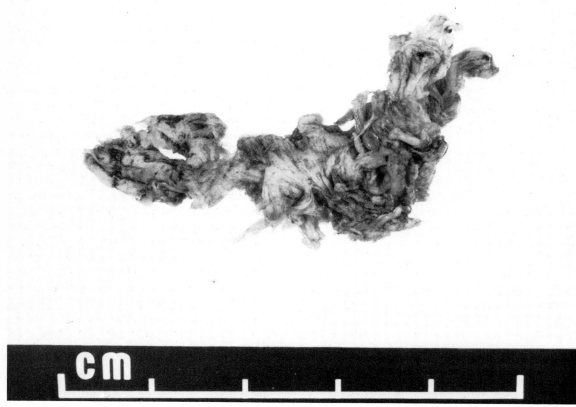

Fig. 12.12   Sequestrated nucleus pulposus.

a diagnostic procedure. If at the time of operation no disc pathology is recognised, and if the vertebral canal is of adequate dimensions, it is preferable to do no more. It is unjustifiable to excise a normal disc, or decompress an adequate canal.

Careful closure and suction drainage is mandatory to avoid haematoma, with its risk of subsequent infection and scar tissue formation.

Chemonucleolysis

Indications

The criteria for chemonucleolysis are the same as those for patients requiring surgery, that is when disc symptoms persist in spite of conservative management (McCulloch, 1977). With reasonable precautions it is a safe procedure and it is often effective (Wiltse, 1983). It is logical to consider chemonucleolysis as the last step in the conservative programme. If there is no indication for surgery there is no place for chemonucleolysis. The radiographic appearance of a generalised disc bulge, not infrequently seen on a CAT scan, is no reason for chemonucleolysis; for success symptoms must correlate with a localised protrusion (Konings et al, 1984). There is no alternative to surgery when massive cauda equina compression affects the bladder, or when the radiculogram suggests migration of a sequestrated fragment.

Technique

General anaesthesia is not necessary, but it probably does make the management of anaphylaxis easier should this complication occur. The procedure is carried out in the operating theatre, with image intensifier control.

The L.4/5 disc is approached from a point adjacent to the iliac crest and 10 centimetres from the mid line. A 15 centimetre number 18 needle is advanced towards the disc space at a 50/60 degree angle. There is a gritty sensation as the needle penetrates the annulus, and the needle is then further advanced into the centre of the nucleus, the position being verified radiographically.

The lumbo-sacral disc space is penetrated with more difficulty. It is approached with a 10 centimetre

needle, number 18, from a point slightly cephalad and medial to that for the L.4/5 disc space. A 15 centimetre number 22 needle is then passed through the lumen of the first needle, with the last two centimetres of the needle bent, so that when it emerges through the first needle, it will curve towards the disc space. It penetrates the annulus into the centre of the nucleus.

If the needle is positioned too far anteriorly, it will cause pain from contact with the nerve root. If posterior, it will impinge on the posterior bony elements. Withdrawal and realignment will provide correct positioning.

Discography verifies the position of the needle, and confirms disruption of the disc, but its volume should be kept to a minimum. A high concentration of radio opaque contrast medium may affect the activity of chymopapain (Naylor et al, 1983) but in vitro tests suggest that after using Hypaque, Conray or Urografin, there is no necessity to delay the therapeutic injection of 2000 to 4000 units of chymopapain. Extravasation of the discographic material through the annular tear into the extra dural space is not a contra-indication to chemonucleolysis. After removing the needles, the patient is placed in the supine position to observe any adverse reactions.

Chemonucleolysis is a potentially life-threatening procedure, for a non-life threatening condition. Major neurological complications have occurred when the enzyme and contrast material have entered the subarachnoid space, with deaths from transverse myelitis and sub arachnoid haemorrhage and cauda equina syndrome. The procedure should be abandoned if the dura is penetrated. The feared complication is anaphylaxis. At particular risk are females who have a sixfold increased incidence of reaction especially those people who have had other allergic phenomena. The severity of reaction is probably reduced by premedication with H.1 and H.2 blockers, blocking histamine's effect — diphenhydramine 50 mg six hourly for 24 hours, and cimetidine 300 mg two hours before anticipated injection. Steroids may be helpful if given in large enough dosage, stabilising the membranes and decreasing permeability. The major problem of anaphylaxis is hypovolaemia, hence preliminary hydration through a large bore IV needle is important.

Anticipation of anaphylaxis lessens the anxiety

should it occur. A large bore IV drip is essential, with blood pressure monitor, intubation facilities, epinephrine 10cc 1:10,000 drawn up in a syringe, diphenhydramine 1 mg/kg, cimetidine 4 mg/kg, steroid 1g, dopamine, bicarbonate and oxygen.

Nausea, itchiness, tingling of the skin, faintness or difficulty in breathing may be the first signs of anaphylaxis, though without warning the pulse and pressure may drop precipitously. Reactions when they occur follow swiftly on the chymopapain injection, but three hours of monitoring is essential.

At the first sign of trouble, anaesthetic is stopped, 100 per cent oxygen is administered, the fluid volume expanded, epinephrine given and acidosis treated. Other drugs are administered as necessary, hydrocortisone, catecholamine, aminophylline, diphenhydramine and cimetidine. The airway is not removed before laryngeal oedema is excluded. Preparation will minimise the morbidity and mortality from anaphylaxis.

There is often immediate relief of sciatic pain (McCulloch, 1980) but quite frequently severe back pain and other leg sensations persist in the early hours after the injection. In a day or two as the back pain settles, the patient is mobilised and returns home.

Chymopapain is more effective than placebo for treatment of patients with a herniated lumbar disc (Javid et al, 1983), and probably better than collagenase.

Chemonucleolysis is probably not as effective in relieving symptoms as surgical excision of the disc (Ejeskar et al, 1983, Crawshaw et al, 1984). Successful chemonucleolysis produces a more rapid recovery than successful surgery (Weir, 1982, Hejna and Sinkora, 1983), but failed chemonucleolysis requiring subsequent surgery carries a poor prognosis. A sequestrated disc is not affected by chemonucleolysis, and this cannot be recognised pre-operatively. It is probably worth removing the disc surgically within a few weeks of the chemonucleolysis if it has obviously failed to relieve the symptoms, rather than delay intervention until chronic pathological changes occur that will not respond to operation.

There is some evidence from increase in the disc space that chemonucleolysis assists regeneration of the intervertebral disc, but this should be viewed with caution. It is possible to produce apparent increases in the disc space when radiographs are not strictly comparable. There is no place for repeat chemonucleolysis because of the increased risk of anaphylaxis.

PROGNOSIS

1. Prognosis — in the short and medium term

It is not possible to predict the ultimate outcome following the first symptoms of a lower lumbar disc lesion. One individual may have disc symptoms from a protrusion and recover with no further trouble. It is more common, however, for symptoms to recur, being precipitated by progressively less severe forces. The first time it may have occurred by lifting a sack of potatoes, and the next with a bucket of coal, and finally by stooping to pick up a piece of paper. The annulus is increasingly less competent to withstand mechanical stress and with each episode a protrusion may progress to an extrusion and finally a sequestration.

The time interval between the first symptoms and final sequestration can be a few days or many years. The pathological process in one patient may have been totally symptomless for years, until a large sequestration suddenly produces disabling symptoms. The history then is measured in days, whilst the pathology may have been present much longer. Another may have had a few days in bed from a protrusion at the age of 20, and finally come to surgery with a sequestration two decades later.

Some present not with episodes of pain, but a steady progression of symptoms over several months, finally requiring surgery at the end of the day. First back pain, then some weeks later ache in the buttock with slight reduction in the straight leg raising. The pain slowly spreads distally over the weeks, with a gradual reduction in straight leg raising, and this is a poor prognostic history.

2. Prognosis — in the long term

The long term prognosis of any disc lesion depends on several factors. Space within the vertebral canal may be at a premium after the development of a posterior annular tear. A protrusion may remain, or extruded nuclear material may fibrose and compromise the canal, and limit the excursion of dura and nerve roots. We have no evidence of annular repair and even though a protrusion may reduce in size, an area of weakness remains, the nucleus degenerates, and the mechanical function of the disc is impaired. It will be less efficient in absorbing energy, and abnormal motion will develop in the intervertebral segment. The speed with which these factors develop is related to the forces exerted on the spine.

Degenerative changes of the borders of the vertebral bodies, and of the apophyseal joints, can encroach into the central canal and the root canal and abnormal motion of the vertebral segment can not only compromise the canal, but also place strain on the structures that resist shear.

Thus a whole series of problems can result from the first disc injury and if we are asked what the future holds for the patient recovering from the first symptom, we just do not know.

With improving health expectations, patients request and require help in the future care of their back after a painful disc lesion. Whether they have recovered at home, required rest in hospital, or had disc excision or chemonucleolysis, they require information about the natural history of disc pathology, and how they can influence it. This can be achieved in the clinic, by physiotherapists in the ward, or in the 'Back School' (page 174). There is no formula for every patient, and the advice is tailored to the individual. It is wise to recommend careful use of the spine, but not at the expense of such limitation of function that disability actually increases. One patient needs restraint, and another encouragement to be more active. There can be a balance between respect for the spine, and a confidence to start to live again which needs to be found with every patient. When encouraged to live within their limitations, the emphasis is on 'live'.

3. Prognosis — after surgery

We are usually asked about the short and long term results of surgical excision of a disc and of chemonucleolysis. Most patients can expect rapid relief of root pain, recovery of mobility, and an early return to work, but they should know that no one can promise success. There are risks to every procedure. Operative fatalities are rare and less with chemonucleolysis. Mortality following excision of an intervertebral disc is 1 in 10,000 (Nelson, 1983) and 1 in 50,000 from anaphylaxis during chemonucleolysis.

Surgical deaths have followed injury to major vessels after penetrating the annulus with a disc extractor. The first sign of such a disaster is not sudden overt haemorrhage, but hypovolaemic shock. It is possible to injure the dura, to damage nerve roots, and to introduce infection, but most patients are made no worse by surgery.

If a patient is no better following surgery, there are but two possibilities. Either the diagnosis was incorrect and should be reviewed, or the operative procedure was inadequate in relieving the root pathology.

One can always expect an appreciable morbidity after even the most properly indicated and competently executed spinal surgery (Connolly, 1983). In fact, the long term results are not encouraging when Selecki and Ness (1982) report 42 per cent of post laminectomy patients unfit to resume their previous occupations, and 22 per cent permanently and totally incapacitated. Naylor (1974) records a continuation of some symptoms in 62 per cent of patients ten years after operation for disc prolapse, and Gurdjian et al (1961) in 71 per cent. Only 30 per cent of those with paresis regain full strength, and only half of the patients have recovery of a sensory deficit (Weber, 1975, 1978). If a disc lesion is not found at operation, the results are worse than non-operative treatment (Hirsch and Machemson, 1963, Nachemson 1976). In fact, one's rate of surgical success is probably related to patient selection rather than technique (Spengler, 1982) and is inversely related to the operative incidence (Rothman, 1972). Verbiest (1977) reported surgical failures due to spinal stenosis in the presence of disc protrusions, and perhaps long term results will improve as the value of decompressing the very narrow vertebral canal is appreciated. We have probably not generally recognised in the past the high incidence of narrowing of the central canal and its frequent trefoil shape in the presence of disc symptoms. It may account for some of the poor surgical results. The dimensions of the vertebral canal are not readily appreciated through the usual limited exposure and iatrogenic scarring of the dura and roots in a limited space, may account for some of the subsequent problems. In addition epidural fibrosis, degenerative changes and abnormal segmental motion can follow disc excision and makes the prognosis inevitably uncertain.

At best, we can relieve the root symptoms, but that spine will always be at risk. In subsequent chapters we are dealing with degenerative syndromes, whose natural history began with a herniated nucleus pulposus.

REFERENCES

Bianco A J 1968 Low back pain and sciatica. Diagnosis and indications for treatment. Journal of Bone and Joint Surgery 50-A: 170–181

Capener N 1933 Alternating sciatic scoliosis. Proceedings of the Royal Society of Medicine 1933: 26: 426–429

Choudhury A R, Taylor J C 1976 Occult lumbar spinal stenosis. Journal of Neurology, Neurosurgery and Psychiatry 40: 506–510

Connolly J F 1983 Does operative treatment of lumbar disc syndrome produce more disability than it prevents? The Nebraska Medical Journa, June 1983: 155–156

Crawshaw C, Frazer A M, Merriam W F, Mulholland R C and Webb J K 1984 A comparison of surgery and chemonucleolysis in the treatment of sciatica; a prospective randomised trial. Spine 9: 195–199

Cyriax J 1978 Dural pain. The Lancet April 29, 1978, P 919–921

Ejeskar A, Nachemson A, Herberts P et al 1983 Surgery versus chemonucleolysis for herniated lumbar discs. A prospective study with random assignment. Clinical Orthopaedics 174: 236–242

Epstein J A, Epstein B S, Levine I 1962. Nerve root compression associated with narrowing of the lumbar spinal canal. Journal of Neurology, Neurosurgery and Psychiatry 25: 165–176

Fries J W, Abodeely D A, Vijungco J G et al 1982 Computed tomography of herniated and extruded nucleus pulposus. Journal of Computer Assisted Tomography 6: 874–877

Frymoyer J W, Hanley E, Howe J et al 1978 Disc excision and spine fusion in the management of lumbar disc disease. A minimum ten year follow up. Spine 3: 1

Grieve G P 1983 Treating backache — a topical comment. Physiotherapy 69: 316

Gurdjian E S, Ostrowski A Z, Hardy W G, Linder D W, Thomas L M 1961. Results of operative treatment of protruded and ruptured lumbar discs. Journal of Neurosurgery 18: 783

Hasue M, Kikuchi S, Sakuyama Y, Ito T 1983 Anatomical study of the inter-relation between nerve roots and their surrounding tissues. Spine 8: 50–58

Haughton V M, Eldevik O P, Magnaes B, Amundsen P 1982 A prospective comparison of computed tomography and myelography in the diagnosis of herniated lumbar discs. Radiology 142: 103–110

Hejna W F, Sinkora G 1983 Chemonucleolysis of herniated lumbar discs. American Family Physician 27: 97–103

Herron L D, Pheasant H C 1983 Bilateral laminotomy and discectomy for segmental lumbar disc disease. Decompression with stability. Spine 8: 86–97

Hirsch C, Nachemson A 1963 The reliability of lumbar disc surgery. Clinical Orthopaedics 29: 189–195

Hudgins W R 1983 The role of microdiscectomy. The Orthopaedic Clinics of North America, 14: 589–603

Javid M J, Nordby E J, Ford L T et al 1983 Safety and efficiency of chymopapain (chymodiactin) in herniated nucleus pulposus with sciatica. Results of a randomised double blind study. JAMA 249: 2489–2494

Kadish L J and Simmons E H 1984 Anomalies of the lumbo-sacral nerve roots: an anatomical investigation and myelographic study. Journal of Bone and Joint Surgery 66-B: 411–416

Konings J G, Williams F J B and Deutman R 1984 The effects of chemonucleolysis as demonstrated by computerised tomography. Journal of Bone and Joint Surgery 66-B: 417–421

McCulloch J A 1977 Chemonucleolysis. Journal of Bone and Joint Surgery 59-B: 45–52

McCulloch J A 1980 Chemonucleolysis: experience with 2000 cases. Clinical Orthopaedics and Related Research 146: 128–135

Mixter W J, Barr J S 1934 Rupture of the intervertebral disc with involvement of the spinal canal. The New England Journal of Medicine 211: 210–215

Nachemson A L 1976 The lumbar spine. An orthopaedic challenge. Spine 1: 59–84

Naylor A 1974 The late results of laminectomy for lumbar disc prolapse. Journal of Bone and Joint Surgery 56-B: 17–29

Naylor A, Earland C and Robinson J 1983 The effect of diagnostic radio-opaque fluids used in discography on chymopapain activity. Spine 8: 875–879

Nelson M 1983. Orthopaedic surgery: Proceedings of the International Symposium on Low Back Pain and Industrial and Social Disablement, P. 91, Back Pain Association.

Paine K W E, Haung P W H 1972 Lumbar disc syndrome. Journal of Neurology 37: 75–82

Patzold U, Haller P, Engelherd P and Weinrich W 1975 Zur fehlhaltung der Lenden Wirbelsanle beim lumbalen. Baldscheiben voofall. Z. Orthop.

Porter R W, Wicks M, Hibbert C 1978 The size of the lumbar spinal canal in the symptomatology of disc lesions. Journal of Bone and Joint Surgery 60-B: 485–487

Porter R W, Miller C 1984. Gravity Induced List. Presented to the International Society for the study of the Lumbar Spine.

Remak E 1881. Deutsch Med Woch 257.

Rothman H R 1972 The patho-physiology of disc degeneration. Clinical Neurosurgery. Proceedings at the Congress of Neurological Surgeons 1972

Rothman R, Wiesel S, Feffer H, Tsournas N, Bell G, Garfin S R, Herkowitz H N, and Booth R E 1984 A study of computer assisted tomography. Volvo Award: Presented to International Society for the Study of the Lumbar Spine, Montreal

Scott J H S 1983 Clinical examination. Ed. John Macleod, sixth edition. Churchill Livingstone. Edinburgh, London, Melbourne and New York

Selecki B R, Ness T D 1982 Multiple operations for a lumbar disc herniation. Australian and New Zealand Journal of Surgery 52: 230

Shenkin H A, Hash C J 1976 A new approach to the surgical treatment of lumbar spondylosis. Journal of Neurosurgery 44: 148–155

Spencer D L, Irwin G S and Miller J A A 1983. Anatomy and significance of fixation of the lumbo-sacral nerve roots in sciatica. Spine 8: 672–679

Spengler D M 1982 Lumbar discectomy: results with limited disc excision and selective foraminotomy. Spine 7: 604–607

Sprangfort E V 1972 The lumbar disc herniation: a computer aided analysis of 2,504 operations. Acta Orthop. Scanda (Suppl. 142) 1

Teplick J G and Haskin M E 1983 CT of the post-operative lumbar spine. Radiological clinics of North America 21: 395–420

Verbiest H 1977 Treatment of idiopathic developmental stenosis of the lumbar vertebral canal. Journal of Bone and Joint Surgery 59–B: 181–188

Weber H 1975 The effect of delayed disc surgery on muscular paresis. Acta Orthop. Scand. 46: 631–642

Weber H 1978 Lumbar disc herniation: evaluation of the total material after 4 years observation. Journal of the Oslo City Hospitals, 28: 91–113

Weber H 1983 Lumbar disc herniation: a controlled prospective study with ten years of observation. Spine 8: 131–140

Weir B 1982 Lumbar discectomy or chemonucleolysis: Pros and Cons. Annals of Surgery 14: 317–329

Williams A L, Haughton V M, Syvertsen A, 1980 Computed tomography in the diagnosis of herniated nucleus pulposus. Radiology 135: 95–99

Williams R 1978 Microlumbar discectomy: A conservative surgical approach to the virgin herniated lumbar disc. Spine 3: 175–182

Wiltse L L 1983 Chemonucleolysis in the treatment of lumbar disc disease. Recent Advances in Orthopaedics. Churchill. Livingstone. Edinburgh, London and New York.

13

Root entrapment syndrome — its pathology, presentation and management

Entrapment of the lumbar nerve root in the root canal (page 29) produces a clinical syndrome distinct from that of the acute disc lesion. In this condition, the root is usually affected by bony and soft tissue encroachment into the root canal and occasionally in the central canal. By contrast, the disc protrusion affects the root in the central canal and uncommonly in the root canal. Though both cause pain in the leg, their presentation and management are distinctly different.

PATHOLOGY

The site of the lesion can be very variable, but the root most commonly involved is the 5th lumbar, probably because of the frequency of degenerative change at L.5/S.1, and the length of the root canal at L.5, inferior to the broad pedicle (Fig. 13.1). The L.4 and L.3 roots are occasionally affected in their root canals. In the central canal the L.5 root can be involved from degenerative change at the L.4/5 disc space (Fig. 18.3, page 147) and the S.1 root anterior to the cranial lip of the upper sacral lamina (Crock, 1981).

The original size of the root canal is variable and must be highly significant. The contents of the root canal also vary, the nerve root and ganglion measuring between 4–7 millimetres in diameter (Weinstein, 1983). Shepperd (1984) measured the difference between the nerve root and the root canal diameter at L.4 and L.5 in fifteen specimens. There was a discrepancy of nil to 5 millimetres. One root in seven of the specimens had an extra-radicular space of less than three millimetres which would be vulnerable to bony and soft tissue encroachment. The root canal will be reduced by a posterior vertebral bar on the infero-lateral border of the body, or by osteophytes

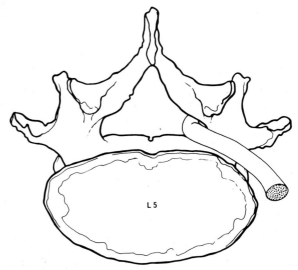

Fig. 13.1 Diagram to show that the L.5 root is vulnerable to the effects of degenerative change along a wide length of the root canal inferior to the broad pedicle.

from the margins of the apophyseal joints (Fig. 13.2). The overhanging medial lip of the superior facet is a common site for 'subarticular entrapment' with the root tightly stretched against the pedicle in the lateral recess. Bony encroachment may follow ossification of spinal ligaments. In spite of the gross degenerative change sometimes encountered in the lower lumbar spine, it is surprising how the nerve root tunnel is always preserved (Fig. 13.3). It may be reduced, but never occluded. If a CT scan should give the impression that the canal is non existent, this is but an artefact of the mathematical display.

Soft tissue involvement of the root canal adds to the bony encroachment. Organisation of an annulus after a disc protrusion, or fibrosis of extruded or sequestrated nucleus, reduces the available space for

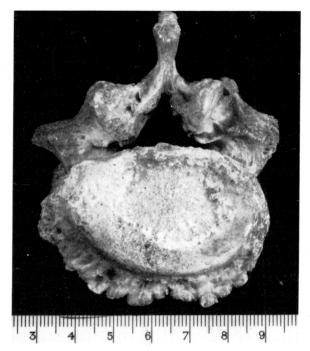

Fig. 13.2 Photograph of fifth lumbar vertebra from below showing marked degenerative change of the vertebral body, posterior vertebral bar formation and osteophytes of the apophyseal joints affecting the root canal bilaterally.

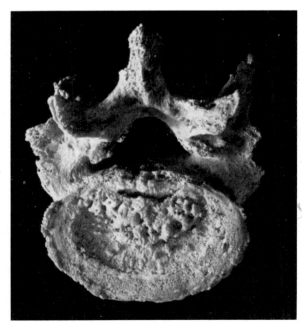

Fig. 13.3 Osteophyte encroaching around the left root canal but the tunnel is preserved.

the root. The posterior longitudinal ligament can thicken, the ligamentum flavum infold (Towme and Reichert, 1931), the apophyseal joint capsule hypertrophy and soft tissue of a lytic pars proliferate until space for the nerve root is at a premium. Venous engorgement in the root canal may critically affect the function of the nerve root.

Segmental movement of the spine adds a dynamic factor (Panjabi et al, 1983). Extension and rotation further reduce available space, and are both limited and painful in this syndrome. It becomes particularly significant when there is posterior or rotational displacement of the vertebra (Fig. 13.4), (Krayenbuhl and Benini, 1979). Degenerative spondylolisthesis can produce the same symptoms (Fig. 13.5). Several dynamic factors can be responsible for symptoms. Postural movement, especially extension, can compromise the root and precipitate symptoms. The activity of walking can produce root symptoms by both intervertebral segmental rotatory movement, and by the epidural venous engorgement associated with exercise. The dynamic factors involved in normal root excursion in activities such as walking and bending, can assume significance in a pathological root.

Just as the tunnel is never occluded, the root is never trapped. There is some excursion, even if at operation the root gives the impression of being tight. The lumbar roots normally have an excursion of a few millimetres limited by proximal and distal attachments (Spencer et al, 1983). These attachments probably make the root vulnerable to traction symptoms in the presence of pathological change. A mobile root in a restricted space will produce root irritation and ischaemia. Friction on a tethered root or anomalous root with limited excursion will have similar results (Kadish and Simmons, 1984). The root then becomes considerably thicker, harder and inelastic from perineural fibrosis.

Wiltse et al (1982) described an unusual cause of root entrapment syndrome when gross displacement of an isthmic spondylolisthesis compresses the L.5 root between the fifth lumbar transverse process and the alar of the sacrum – 'the far out syndrome'.

There are many pathological changes that can cause lumbar root pain in the middle aged and older patient. The most common site of these changes is in the root canal, related to disc pathology of a previous decade.

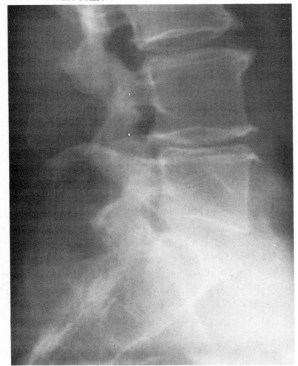

Fig. 13.4A Radiograph of a patient with root entrapment syndrome whose pain was related to extension and rotation of the spine. There is disc degeneration at L.4/5 with posterior osteophyte formation and some displacement.

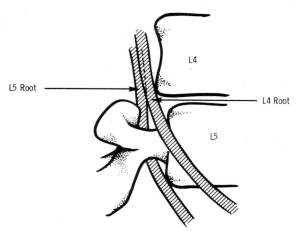

Fig. 13.4B Diagram to show how the L.4 root is affected by posterior or rotational vertebral displacement.

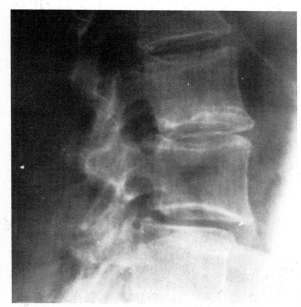

Fig. 13.5 Lateral radiograph of a patient with root pain. Degenerative spondylolisthesis at L.4/5 is associated with reduction of space in the root canal.

CLINICAL PRESENTATION

Though the pain from root entrapment is in the same distribution as the sciatica from a disc lesion, from the buttock, thigh, calf to the foot, its character is different. It is described as a severe pain often unremitting day and night. Whilst the pain from a disc is frequently relieved by lying down, this pain is so troublesome at night that the patient will walk about. Sitting is uncomfortable, driving far impossible, as though the whole length of the sciatic nerve is over-sensitive. Unlike root pain of disc origin it is unaffected by coughing and sneezing.

The periodicity of the pain is variable. One patient may experience constant severe pain, and present at the consulting room after many sleepless nights. Another may have mild pain with episodes of severe pain in relation to posture, especially to sitting or standing for long. Another may say that walking is the main cause of pain. If walking only produces pain, one should suspect a vascular component, either venous engorgement of the root canal or arterial insufficiency of the root.

The past history is also variable. There has usually been previous disc pathology, but the previous disc symptoms may have been either classical, with root pain, or have produced only back pain; they may even have been entirely occult. The degree of original disc symptoms years before depends much on the size of the central vertebral canal. There may have been no symptoms at all from a disc protrusion into a wide domeshaped central canal, but with disc space narrowing over the years, bony and soft tissue degeneration and perhaps slight vertebral displacement, the root becomes compromised. The very first symptom of the silent lesion years before is now severe root pain from root canal entrapment.

The progress of the root pain once it has developed is unpredictable. It can develop and subside in weeks, months or years, and patients may therefore present with long or short histories. It has no typical pattern, sometimes being severe and gradually resolving, and at other times getting steadily worse, requiring surgery.

The abnormal signs are generally few. In a series of 249 patients, we found that 32 per cent could reach down to touch the floor with straight knees. Lumbar extension however was considered to be full in only 12 per cent. SLR was eighty degrees or more in 74 per cent. Reflexes were normal in 84 per cent, sensation normal in 82 per cent, and muscle wasting and weakness recorded in less than 5 per cent. Only one-third of Getty's patients with root entrapment (1981) had significant restriction of straight leg raising, and this was similarly recorded by Macnab (1977). For many patients with little to find clinically, the diagnosis begs therefore a good history. Most patients have some radiological evidence of degenerative change, reduction of L.5/S.1 disc space being the most consistent finding. Central canal measurements are little different from the general population (Table 11.1, page 87). There is a greater incidence of abnormal neurological signs in those patients who have had previous surgery, and in those referred for surgery from other units because of the intensity and duration of root symptoms.

In expert hands, electromyography can provide objective evidence of impaired root function and it will sometimes identify the root affected (Leyshon et al, 1980). Other studies with electromyography have not confirmed the ability of this investigation to predict which nerve roots are responsible for symptoms (Merriam et al, 1982), probably because of the variable anatomy of root innervation.

Electrodiagnostic methods can complement other investigations and help in the overall evaluation but probably have limited value, especially after previous laminectomy (Eisen and Hoirch, 1983).

Radiculography has a poor sensitivity for root entrapment syndrome (Euinton et al, 1984) but it will exclude other pathology in the severely disabled patient.

CT scan is advisable if surgery is being seriously considered. Bony encroachment may of course not be the cause of the symptoms but CT scan is a valuable adjunct to surgery (Fig. 13.6).

The absence of fat in the root canal and in the lateral recess can be demonstrated by nuclear magnetic resonance, and will support the diagnosis of root entrapment syndrome (Crawshaw et al, 1984).

MANAGEMENT

Most patients presenting to an orthopaedic surgeon with root entrapment syndrome can be managed by a

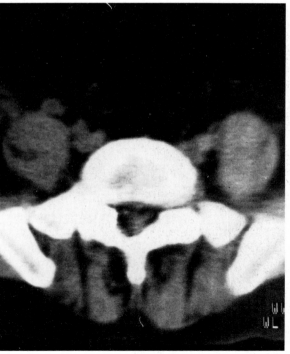

Fig. 13.6 CT scan of a patient with severe pain in a lumbar root distribution, showing a narrow canal and overhanging facet.

careful explanation of the cause of pain, and advice. 81 per cent of our patients were managed in this way (Porter and Hibbert, 1984). They certainly need to be given time to discuss the probable cause of the pain, and to understand that if aggravating factors can be avoided, it will probably settle. If sitting for long and standing increase the symptoms, the position should be quickly changed. The mechanical stress on the spine should be kept to a minimum, and if this is not understood, it is reinforced with a back school programme. They are told that symptoms will probably remain for a long time, but will reduce in intensity and eventually settle.

Of our patients with root entrapment 187 described their symptoms after two years. Three-quarters of them still had some root pain, but it was less troublesome and only 12 per cent had either returned in those two years or sought help elsewhere.

For some patients the pain is so intense it is not reasonable to offer advice only. It is difficult to obtain statistical evidence that an epidural injection is better than placebo (Klenerman et al, 1984), but there is strong circumstantial evidence that this is perhaps the best indication for an epidural. Although it may not always be effective, many patients admit that the epidural is the start of improvement, whilst others obtain immediate and complete relief of pain. 40 cc of normal saline, with 2 cc of steroid and local anaesthetic, injected epidurally at the level of the lesion, can produce good results. After two years, more of our patients who had had epidurals were free of pain than those untreated and they were those with most severe symptoms. The results were not statistically significant. For a few patients, surgical decompression of the root canal is essential. Careful patient selection is vital to obtain a good result. The diagnosis must be correct, the symptoms sufficiently severe, and not resolving by conservative means. The diagnosis can be difficult, and supplementary evidence from investigations is always welcome. Myelography is generally unhelpful, the lesion being too far lateral to be detected. EMGs may support the clinical diagnosis and a CT scan is imperative, especially if there has been previous surgery. It is most helpful in demonstrating the bony contours of the central and root canal, and the degree of encroachment by bone and ligamentum flavum. When facet degenerative change is a significant factor, the extent of undercutting of the superior facet can be predicted.

How can we assess the severity of the pain? We can only observe the patient's behaviour in response to pain, and unfortunately the degree of the root pathology is not at all related to the patient's behaviour to that pathology. Exaggerated signs are associated with exaggerated symptoms. The root pathology may not be as gross as the symptoms suggest, and the subsequent results of surgery a disappointment. In a condition where symptoms outweigh the abnormal signs, a pre-operative psychological assessment is a useful supplement to the clinical examination. It may indicate an abnormal profile with a poor prognosis.

Before considering surgery, there should also be an adequate period of observation over several weeks lest the condition will resolve either naturally or with the help of one or more epidural injections. When the diagnosis is clear, the pain severe and of long duration, when it is not settling and there is no evidence of exaggeration, surgical decompression of the root can be rewarding. Getty recorded early relief of leg pain in 68 per cent of his operated patients (1981).

Decompression of the root requires adequate exposure of the root over the length at risk. (Scoville and Corkhill, 1973). The site of compression may be suspected pre-operatively by conventional radiography, by CT scan, or occasionally by myelography. Electrical studies may identify the root. The area is exposed surgically, and the root followed proximally and distally until there is no question at all that it is free and mobile. There is sometimes, however, uncertainty about the area of pathology, and about the root which is involved, and it may be necessary to explore the lower lumbar central canal and two root canals fairly extensively. The confidence with which one views the investigations will determine the extent of surgical exploration. Many feel that a wide decompression is generally necessary, removing the spinous process and laminae at L.5, occasionally at L.4 if the 4th lumbar root is suspect, and following the L.5 root well into the root canal undercutting the lamina to ensure complete freedom for the root. The L.5 root may be obviously thickened and tough with perineural fibrosis, and there is then no doubt about the root involved. Bony hypertrophy in the 5th lumbar root canal should not cause us to automatically suspect that root. The S.1 root may be the cause of the symptoms, and removal of the upper sacral lamina may, in fact, reveal compression under the cranial lip.

Others more confident of the site of the lesion may be happy to perform a limited decompression, removing the window of lamina and part of the apophyseal joint, undercutting the lamina and removing ligamentum flavum (Getty et al, 1981). There are obvious advantages in a more limited exposure provided the decompression is adequate. Most patients experience early post-operative relief of their leg pain but not a few have persisting symptoms of varying degree, perhaps the result of irreversible root pathology.

REFERENCES

Crawshaw C, Kean D M, Mulholland R C, Worthington B S, Finlay D, Hawkes R C, Gyngell M and Moore W S 1984 The use of nuclear magnetic resonance in the diagnosis of lateral canal entrapment.

Crock H V 1981 Normal and pathological anatomy of the lumbar spinal nerve root canals. Journal of Bone and Joint Surgery 63-B: 487-490

Eisen N A, Hoirch M 1983 The electrodiagnostic evaluation of spinal root lesions. Spine 8: 98-106

Euinton H A, Locke T J, Barrington N A, Getty C J M and Davies G K 1984 Radiological diagnosis of bony entrapment of lumbar nerve roots using water soluble radiculography. Presented to the International Society for the Study of the Lumbar Spine, Montreal

Getty C J M, Johnson J R, Kirwan E O'G, Sullivan M F 1981 Partial undercutting facetectomy for bony entrapment of the lumbar nerve root. Journal of Bone and Joint Surgery 63-B: 330-335

Kadish L J and Simmons E H 1984 Anomalies of the lumbosacral nerve roots: an anatomical investigation and myelographic study. Journal of Bone and Joint Surgery. 66-B: 411-416.

Klenerman L, Greenwood R, Davenport H T, White D C, Peskett S 1984 Lumbar epidural injections in the treatment of sciatica. British Journal of Rheumatology 23: 35-38

Krayenbuhl H, Benini A 1979 Die enge des recessus lateralis im lumalen bereich der wirbelsaule als ursa che der nervenwurzelkompression bei bandscheibenvers chamlerung. Z. Orthop. 117: 167-171

Leyshon A, Kirwan E O'G, Wynn Parry C B 1980 Is it nerve root pain? Journal of Bone and Joint Surgery 62-B: 119

Macnab I 1977 Backache. Baltimore. Williams and Wilkins Co. 1977

Merriam W F, Smith N J, Mulholland R C 1982 Lumbar spinal stenosis. British Medical Journal 285: 515

Panjabi M M, Takata K, Goel U K, 1983 Kinematics of lumbar intervertebral foramen. Spine 8: 348-357

Porter R W, Hibbert C, Evans C 1984 The natural history of root entrapment syndrome Spine 9: 418-422

Scoville W B, Corkhill G 1973 Lumbar disc surgery: technique of radical removal and early mobilisation. Journal of Neurosurgery 39: 265-269

Shepperd J A N 1984 Anatomy of the L.4/L.5 and S.1 nerve roots and their associated thecal sheaths: cadaver studies. Personal communication

Spencer D L, Irwin G S and Miller J A A 1983 Anatomy and significance of fixation of the lumbosacral nerve roots in sciatica. Spine 8: 672-679

Towme E B, Reichert F L 1931 Compression of the lumbosacral roots of the spinal cord by thickened ligamenta flava. Annals of Surgery 94: 327-336

Weinstein P R 1983 Diagnosis and management of lumbar spinal stenosis. Clinical Neurosurgery 30: 677-697

Wiltse L, Glenn W, Spencer C, Porter I and Guyer R 1982. Alar transverse process impingement of the L.5 spinal nerve (The Far Out syndrome). Presented to the International Society for the Study of the Lumbar Spine, Toronto.

14

Neurogenic claudication — its clinical presentation, differential diagnosis, pathology and management

The term 'claudication of the spinal cord' was first used by DeJerine (1911) when describing three patients with claudication symptoms but normal peripheral pulses. Van Gelderen (1948) reported a patient with symptoms of lumbar root compression which appeared on walking and was relieved by rest, which he thought was due to thickening of the ligamentum flavum. Bergmark (1950) described 'intermittent spinal claudication' attributing a neurospinal origin to the walking pains of two patients. It was Verbiest in 1954 who recognised that structural narrowing of the vertebral canal could compress the cauda equina, and produce claudication symptoms, and since that time there have been numerous publications on the subject (Gathier, 1959, Brish et al, 1964, Dyck and Doyle, 1977, Bowen et al, 1978, Blau and Logue, 1978).

CLINICAL PRESENTATION

This intriguing syndrome usually affects men over 50 years of age, who have been heavy manual workers. They complain of discomfort in the legs when walking, affecting both legs equally, usually in the thighs, calves and feet. Describing the discomfort is difficult, but they describe the legs as feeling 'heavy' or 'tired', as though it is difficult to drag one leg after another. One man says his legs felt like those of a deep sea diver, another as though he had cricket pads on his legs. There is usually a threshold distance when the discomfort develops, and a tolerance when they have to stop, and the tolerance is about twice the threshold. The distance can vary during the day, from one day to the next, and even during one stretch of walking. The second period of walking can be longer than the first after a short rest. Often they find they

gradually reduce the walking speed and stoop forwards until they finally stop — the stoop test (Dyck, 1979) (Fig. 14.1). They will lean forwards on a wall, or stoop forwards and tie up a shoelace to save embarrassment, and after a few minutes the feeling in the legs recovers sufficiently for them to start walking again. The flexed position seems to relieve the

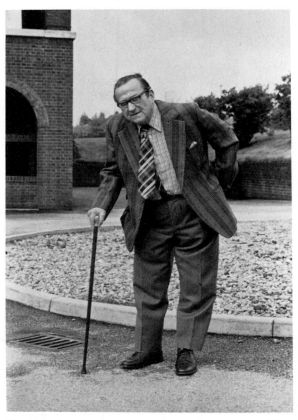

Fig. 14.1 A patient with neurogenic claudication stops walking because of discomfort in the legs and stoops forwards to relieve the symptoms.

discomfort and for that reason they may be able to walk better up a hill leaning forwards, than down a hill leaning back. Extending the spine in the standing position can precipitate symptoms in the severely disabled patient. They say they can cycle for miles and can climb a ladder and stairs, but not come down stairs easily. As the condition progresses, the walking distance reduces sometimes to only 20 yards. It is probably not neurogenic claudication if a man can walk more than a mile at a reasonable pace without having to stop.

Nights are usually troublesome, with sleep being disturbed by restless legs and night cramps. They disturb their wives, and will often get up and walk about at night.

Back pain is a common but not an invariable accompaniment. There is usually a long history of back pain, sometimes with previous surgery, and claudication symptoms for a number of years before they seek help.

Apart from the spinal posture, the examination is remarkable for its lack of gross abnormality. They may be able to flex well forward with extended knees though lumbar extension is usually absent. In fact, it may be difficult to even stand erect and these patients adopt a 'Simian stance' (Simkin, 1982), with hips and knees slightly flexed (Fig. 14.2). This can be corrected with an effort, but it quickly returns as they relax. If this posture is not present at rest, it tends to develop with walking, the patient gradually stooping further forward until he has to stop.

The 'stoop-test' makes use of this phenomenon in diagnosing claudication of neurogenic origin, the leg symptoms being relieved by stooping forwards at the point of walking tolerance, and returning by standing upright again. The lumbar spine is often tender over several segments. S.L.R. is generally full, the reflexes normal, the power and sensation also normal. It has been suggested that re-examination after excercise alters the neurological examination but this is not our experience. The peripheral circulation is normal but not infrequently arterial disease will co-exist. A treadmill enables us to establish an objective record of walking pain, noting the distance at which symptoms develop, the distribution of discomfort, the speed of walking, the changing posture, and the tolerance (Fig. 14.3). The impression gained from the patient's history can be completely different from an objective assessment of walking. When measuring a response to treatment, a treadmill in invaluable.

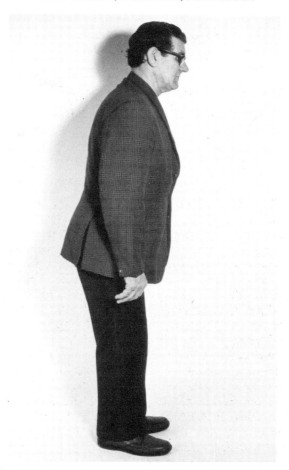

Fig. 14.2   The typical posture of a patient with neurogenic claudication standing with flexed hips and knees, the Simian stance.

A plain radiograph may raise the suspicion of a shallow vertebral canal and perhaps show a degenerative spondylolisthesis, present in half the men with neurogenic claudication. A myelogram is essential to confirm the diagnosis. It will show one or several segmental filling defects, or even a complete block (Fig. 14.4). The lack of space in the central canal can make injection of the contrast medium very difficult, and the myelogram may have to be abandoned at the lower lumbar level (Williams, 1975, Ehni, 1969). When myelography is difficult, epidural venography will show the extent of the stenosis (Bestawros et al, 1979).

CT complements radiculography (Black et al, 1982) demonstrating the canal's mid sagittal diameter, cross sectional area and shape. We must examine a longer

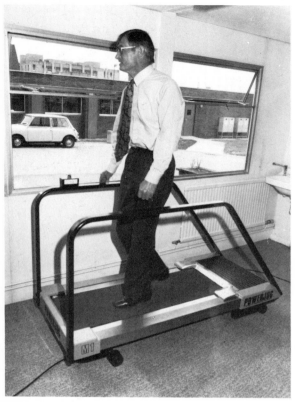

Fig. 14.3 A treadmill provides an objective assessment of walking distance and posture.

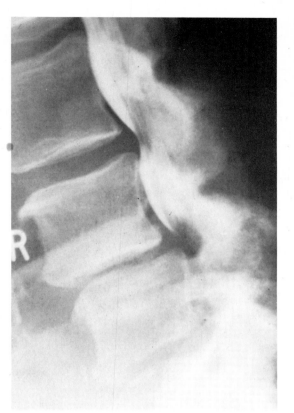

Fig. 14.4 A radiograph of a 63 year old man with neurogenic claudication showing partial occlusion of the metrizamide column at L.3/4 and a complete block at L.4/5, the site of a degenerative spondylolisthesis.

segment of canal than the standard L.3 to S.1 for disc problems, increasing the radiation dose, but this is outweighed by its advantages. Bony encroachment, thickened ligamentum flavum and disc material may be evident. The extent of undercutting facetectomy can be predicted.

Ultrasound measurements confirm a reduced mid sagittal diameter of the vertebral canal.57 per cent of our patients with neurogenic claudication had measurements below the tenth percentile and 42 per cent below the fifth percentile. A narrow canal supports the diagnosis, but obviously narrow canals exist without neurogenic claudication symptoms. A wide canal is incompatible with the diagnosis.

DIFFERENTIAL DIAGNOSIS

1. Intermittent claudication, a phrase coined by Charcot in 1858 to describe ischaemic pain from peripheral vascular disease, is difficult to distinguish from neurogenic claudication by the history alone. It is not affected by posture, and the patient does not find himself stooping forwards the further he walks. He finds climbing hills worse than descending them, and he can neither cycle nor walk. The bicycle test of van Gelderen (1948) modified by Dyck and Doyle (1977) is helpful in differentiating between these two types of claudication. The patient is asked to cycle with the spine first extended and then flexed. The distance is the same in intermittent claudication whilst in neurogenic claudication the flexed position allows greater exercise tolerance (Fig. 14.5). His walking threshold and tolerance are generally much the same from one day to the next. One leg may be more affected than the other, and perhaps only the calves. These, however, are generalisations, and in practice the difference between the two is not always straightforward. Impalpable peripheral pulses and

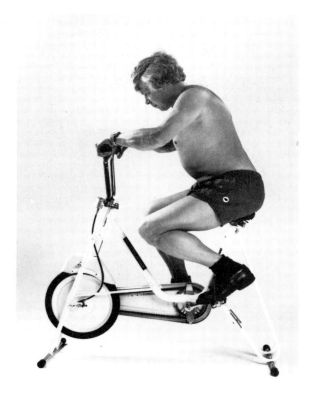

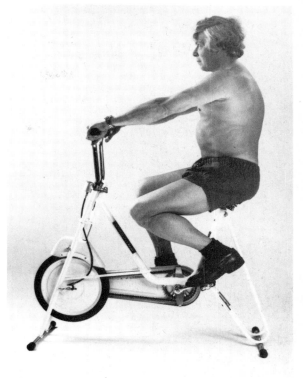

Fig. 14.5A A patient with neurogenic claudication can cycle without pain if the spine is flexed.

Fig. 14.5B Symptoms develop in the legs when the patient with neurogenic claudication cycles in the upright position. The symptoms of intermittent claudication are not affected by cycling posture.

femoral bruits will suggest peripheral vascular disease. If clinical examination is difficult, a doppler scan may be more objective, but it can take an arteriogram to be certain of the relative importance of the peripheral arterial circulation. Cerebral somato-sensory evoked potentials after walking may help to differentiate neurogenic from vascular intermittent claudication (Larson and Milwarkee, 1983). To confuse the issue, intermittent claudication and neurogenic claudication may coexist (Johansson et al, 1982).

2. Lamerton et al (1983) described sciatic claudication, an insufficiency of the inferior gluteal artery producing claudication in a sciatic distribution from ischaemia of the sciatic nerve. The claudication is in a root distribution but spinal examination and myelography are normal. It is an important condition to recognise. Endarterectomy of the aorto-iliac segments can relieve the symptoms, whilst an arterial

graft by disturbing the inferior gluteal artery and its anastomoses, will be ineffective.

3. Referred pain from the lower lumbar region in the buttocks and thighs, even to the upper calves, can be aggravated by walking. 18 per cent of Crock's patients with isolated lumbar disc resorption (Venner and Crock, 1981) had increasing leg pain or paraesthesia on walking distances up to 500 yards. We can recognise referred pain from its proximal distribution not beyond the upper calves, and its presence in activities other than walking. A normal myelogram is compatible with referred pain, but not with neurogenic claudication.

4. Some types of root pain and multiple root pathology are made worse by walking (Jayson and Nelson, 1979), probably if segmental instability is a factor in producing the root symptoms, and if venous engorgement contributes to restriction of space in the root canal. There may be little or no pain at rest, but

walking precipitates unilateral leg pain with a variable threshold and tolerance which is relieved by stopping and leaning forwards. Root claudication may be the remaining symptom after a classical disc protrusion has settled down, or it may occur in the older patient with root entrapment from lateral bony stenosis.

5. Claudication pain is sometimes a symptom of distress. Abnormal behaviour patterns are common in patients who have a long history of back pain, and not infrequently a symptom inappropriate to the underlying organic problem in the spine, is pain in the legs when walking. There are usually inappropriate signs also.

Case history

Mrs J.M., a 45 year old housewife, complained of pain in both legs when walking, which had gradually developed over the past five years, limiting her walking distance to 30 yards. She had no previous history of back pain, but did have back pain now, interfering with housework. She found climbing stairs and going up a slope difficult. She slept fairly well. She was a little overweight. She found it difficult to get up from a chair, and walked across the room slowly and awkwardly. Flexion and extension of the lumbar spine were both somewhat limited. Reflexes and motor power were normal. She had bounding peripheral pulses. There were six inappropriate signs. Axial loading and simulated rotation both gave pain in the lower lumbar region. There was widespread tenderness, discomfort to light squeezing of the lumbar skin, straight leg raising was resisted and there was non-dermatomal sensory loss. Ultrasound measurements of the vertebral canal were below the tenth percentile, and lest a genuine spinal stenosis was missed she had a myelogram. It was normal. She was told that there was no evidence of a serious disorder causing her symptoms, that she would get better rather than worse, but she wept at the thought of not being offered active treatment.

6. It is difficult to accurately assess the claudicating patient who also has a litigation problem. One can exclude a peripheral vascular lesion, and if the myelogram is normal, exclude neurogenic claudication. An equivocal myelogram is a problem. Although the diagnosis would be suspect with more than one inappropriate sign, these signs may mask a genuine underlying problem. Litigation can so confuse the issue, that it may not be possible to decide how much of the symptoms are organic, and whether the organic element of the leg pain is neurogenic claudication, multiple root pathology, or referred pain.

7. There are other less common causes of claudication pain. Venous claudication can follow thrombosis before the colateral circulation takes over,

the increased venous pressure affecting the perfusion pressure. The pain brought on by exercise is only relieved as the leg is elevated.

Myxoedema claudication results from the limited potential of muscle to increase its metabolism with exercise. Pulses are normal. Symptoms are completely relieved by treating the hypothyroidism.

Rarely a localised deep arterio venous fistula will present with aching and pain in the legs aggravated by exercise and standing. The muscle cannot respond to exercise by significantly increasing its arterial flow. Usually congenital or acquired fistulae demonstrate obviously dilated veins, sometimes pulsatile, a swelling, a bruit, distal venous insufficiency and hemi hypertrophy in the young.

It is not difficult to recognise degenerative changes of the weight bearing joints as a cause of ambulatory leg pain.

PATHOLOGY

Verbiest (1954) recognised that neurogenic claudication was associated with a shallow vertebral canal. In fact the term 'spinal stenosis' has unfortunately become synonymous with neurogenic claudication, when in fact a shallow canal is only one factor in the pathology. Symptoms develop after middle life but there is no evidence that the vertebral canal becomes narrower with age. There can be a little encroachment into the canal from hypertrophy of the apophyseal joints and marginal osteophyte formation, but this is more into the root canal than the central canal. Also posterior vertebral bar formation on the lower and upper posterior margins of the vertebral bodies can reduce the sagittal diameter to some degree. In general, however, the central canal retains the same cross sectional diameter throughout life. An individual with spinal stenosis and neurogenic claudication has therefore had a narrow canal for many years before the development of leg symptoms (Salibi, 1976, Ami Hood and Weigl, 1983, Critchley, 1982) and many patients with stenotic canals never have claudication pain. The canal is therefore but one factor in the pathology.

A second factor is degenerative disease of the lumbar spine associated with heavy manual work. The majority of patients with neurogenic claudication have been involved in heavy work. Few have been sedentary workers. It would seem that the accumulative effects of the mechanical stress of labouring work plays a part in pathology rather than the degenerative process from one disc insult in the earlier life of a sedentary worker.

The high male incidence of nine to one may be due to heavier manual work, or indicate that hormonal factors are significant.

Vertebral displacement with an intact neural arch will critically narrow an already small canal (Fig. 14.6, 14.7). Degenerative spondylolisthesis effectively reduces the canal size at the level of displacement (Rosenberg, 1976, Wilson and Brill, 1977). Although degenerative spondylolisthesis is more common in women, half of the men with neurogenic claudication in our series had a degenerative spondylolisthesis (Porter and Hibbert, 1983). Women with degenerative displacement rarely develop claudication symptoms (Fig. 14.8).

Neurogenic claudication must be very unusual in children but Birkensfield and Kasdon (1978)

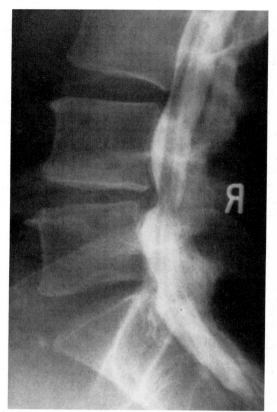

Fig. 14.7 Radiculogram of a 61 year old man with neurogenic claudication. There is an anterior filling defect at L.3/4 associated with some posterior and rotational vertebral displacement. The clear outline of the roots of the cauda equina ('a canal full of roots') suggests that the cross sectional area of the canal is reduced by a trefoil configuration.

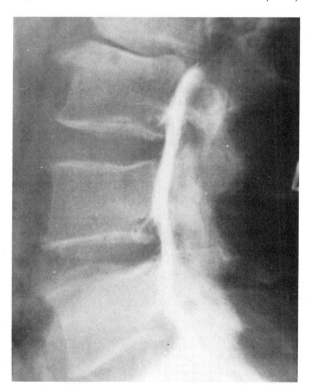

Fig. 14.6 A lateral radiograph of a 58 year old man with neurogenic claudication. The vertebral canal is particularly narrow and is completely blocked at L.2/3 level, the site of disc degeneration and retrospondylolisthesis.

described it in two adolescent boys with congenital lumbar ridges producing ventral defects on myelography.

Symptoms are probably the result of inadequate oxygenation of the cauda equina, but the mechanism is at present purely speculative. There may be arterial ischaemia or venous engorgement, which just permits adequate nerve function at rest, but inadequate function during exercise. The fact that patients are generally over fifty years of age when arteriosclerosis is becoming more common, is compatible with an ischaemic component to the pathology. Many claudicating patients have a stenosis at L.3/4 level. This may have a neuro-ischaemic explanation. The proximal third of the cauda equina is an area at risk, being supplied by an astomosis of both proximal and distal radicular arteries. If the supply is just adequate

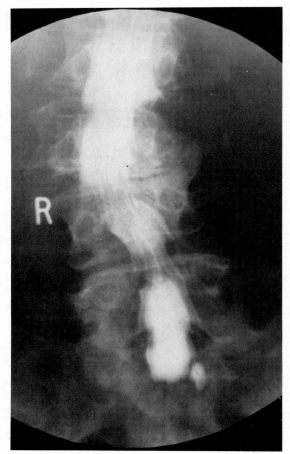

Fig. 14.8A A radiculogram of a 68 year old woman with neurogenic claudication showing occlusion of the metrizamide column at L.4/5 associated with a structural lumbar scoliosis.

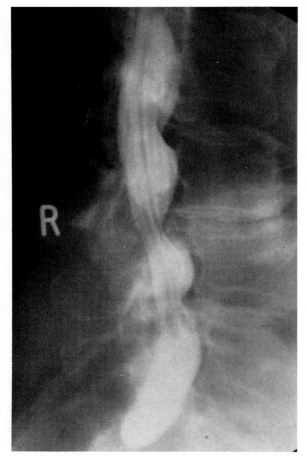

Fig. 14.8B Her lateral radiculogram shows multiple filling defects.

for its needs (Domminisse, 1976), then deprivation could precipitate claudication symptoms at this level.

Fifty years ago, Reichert et al described ischaemia of the spinal cord due to arteriosclerotic involvement of the lumbar arteries, giving weakness of the lower limbs on exertion. He noted similar temporary weakness in dogs by ligation of the lumbar artery. Cauda equina ischaemia may have a similar mechanism.

There is probably localised vasodilatation of the radicular arteries in response to exercise. Exercising the single limb of a mouse will produce vasodilatation of the ipsilateral region of the spinal cord (Blau and Rushworth, 1958). In addition, the selective paralysis in poliomyelitis is probably related to the vasodilatation of the anterior horn in response to

muscular activity in the pre-paralytic stage of the disease (Buchthal, 1949). Should the vessels of the cauda equina likewise dilate with exercise, they will be vulnerable to ischaemia if space is at a premium.

The ischaemic factor seems to be particularly relevant in some patients.

Case history

Mr S.R., a salesman, had surgery for coarctation of the aorta at 27 years of age. He had a brachial artery pressure of 230/130 with delayed low velocity femoral pulses, and impalpable peripheral pulses. The aorta distal to the thoracic coarctation was 1 cm diameter and hypoplastic. Two cm of the coarctation were removed with relief of his fatigue symptoms and headaches. A lumbar disc was excised four years later, and at the age of 39 he had claudication symptoms. A spinal decompression then relieved the leg symptoms only temporarily, and now at 43 years of age his walking tolerance is only 150 yards. An arteriogram shows competence of the aorto-iliac, femoral and popliteal segments (Fig. 14.9). It is unusual for neurogenic claudication to present in the fourth decade, and especially in a sedentary worker. The aortic and lumbar disc pathology with iatrogenic scarring, probably combined to produce critical cauda equina ischaemia with exercise.

A vascular steal syndrome could explain the claudication symptoms of some patients with claudication and Paget's disease, when the vertebral canal may not appear significantly narrow (Ravichandran, 1981, Douglas et al, 1981, Herzberg and Bayliss, 1980).

Iatrogenic neurogenic claudication can follow spinal surgery more so after a spinal fusion than discectomy. The patient is at risk whose developmentally narrow canal is fused. It was previously thought that bony ingrowth from the posterior fusion mass compromised the canal causing symptoms, but it is more likely that symptoms arise at the segment proximal to the fusion. It can become unstable, and the narrow canal, segmental instability, and ischaemia from iatrogenic scarring combine to produce symptoms.

Claudication is related to the dynamic activity of walking. There are probably three processes caused by walking which precipitate symptoms in a cauda equina already deprived and vulnerable. Segmental rotation which accompanies walking, especially with segmental instability, will reduce the available space in an already narrow canal. Secondly, the increased venous return from the exercising lower limbs will be accompanied by engorgement of the pelvic veins and of Batson's venous plexus, reducing the available space for the cauda equina. Thirdly, the arterial system of the cauda equina must respond to the increasing demands of exercise, and may do so inadequately when space is limited. Nutriments fail to reach the nerve roots, metabolites are not removed, and function is affected. The first process is probably the most critical because it is not the exercise of the lower limbs that produces the symptoms, but rather the torque and posture of the spine at the time of that exercise. A fourth mechanism may be responsible if there exists a lumbar artery shunt (page 26). In health, the intraosseous arterial branches of the lumbar arteries may vasoconstrict and shunt blood to the radicular branch, during the activity of walking or running. If there is already incipient ischaemia of the nerve roots from restricted space in the vertebral canal, and if in addition the vertebral shunt should fail as a result of bony degenerative pathology, neurogenic claudication symptoms would develop in times of physiological stress.

As yet, we do not know how important is the cerebrospinal fluid in the normal function of the cauda equina. It is possible that this is the key to the mechanism of the symptoms of neurogenic claudication (Porter, 1982). The cauda equina probably needs to be bathed in a free circulation of cerebrospinal fluid for its nutrition for removal of metabolites, and for insulation. When the fluid is deficient from reduced space in the canal, and especially when there is a closed sac of fluid distally, the circulation will be deficient. Magnaes (1982) was able to record a high cerebral spinal fluid pressure in claudicating patients caudal to a stenosed segment and related to posture. One can imagine a claudicating patient stopping after a few hundred yards, leaning forwards on a wall for a minute, and as the fluid above the stenosis is permitted to exchange with the closed sac below, the discomfort rapidly clears from the legs. It is interesting that neurogenic claudication does not usually occur from stenosis at L.5/S.1 alone. It is usually from segmental narrowing at the two or three more proximal segments which permits a closed sac of dura distally. If the sac is too large from stenosis at the thoraco lumbar level,

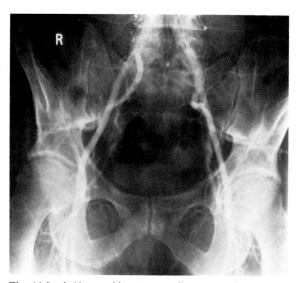

Fig. 14.9 A 43 year old man unusually young to have symptoms of neurogenic claudication. His decompression at L.4/5 only temporarily relieved his symptoms. The aortic and femoral segments are patent on arteriography.

claudication symptoms are rare. Although L.3/4 interspace is the most common level of stenosis in neurogenic claudication (Schatzker and Pennal, 1968, and Weisz, 1983), it is still possible for a large disc protrusion at L.5/S.1 to produce the same symptoms.

Case report

Mr J.J. was a 27 year old cricketer who developed back pain and bilateral leg pains over a six month period. His main concern was discomfort in both legs walking, which stopped him at 100 yards. S.L.R. was 90/40. A myelogram showed a central disc lesion at L.5/S.1 with an extensive distal dural sac (Fig. 14.10). A month after excising the disc and decompressing the canal, his walking distance was unlimited. The long closed sac phenomenon could account for the claudication symptoms.

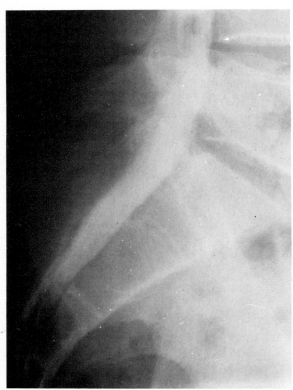

Fig. 14.10 Lateral radiculogram of a 27 year old cricketer who developed a central disc protrusion at L.5/S.1 producing bilateral claudication symptoms. There is an extensive distal dural sac.

MANAGEMENT

Patients with neurogenic claudication are either offered surgical decompression, or are advised to live with their symptoms. If symptoms are not too severe,

or if surgery is contra-indicated, simple reduction of activities, alteration of job, together with instruction on the correct postures for lifting and carrying, may enable the patients to live within their limitations (Jayson and Nelson, 1979). Once the syndrome is well established, however, conservative management rarely improves the quality of life (Ami Hood and Weigl, 1983).

It is our policy to offer a course of Calcitonin to patients with neurogenic claudication. The beneficial effect of Calcitonin on the paraperesis of patients with spinal Paget's disease was noted by Walpin and Singer, 1979, Herzberg and Bayliss, 1980, Douglas et al, 1981, Ravichandran, 1981. Many of their patients,

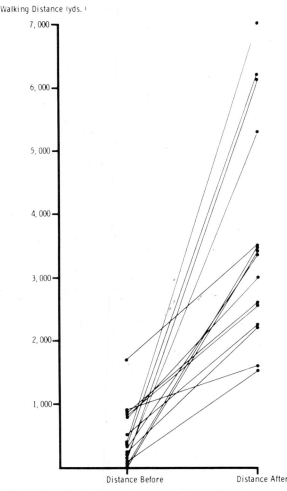

Fig. 14.11 Graph to show improvement in walking distance of 15 patients whose neurogenic claudication was treated with calcitonin.

besides losing the Paget's pain, also found that their walking improved suddenly and dramatically.

It is essential to exclude other causes of claudication — vascular disease, referred pain, multiple root pathology, and claudication as a sign of distress. We give 100 units of calcitonin intramuscularly four times a week for four weeks. If the walking distance has not improved by the fourth week, the drug is discontinued, but if there is some improvement, the regime is continued for a further four weeks (Fig. 14.11). Calcitonin engenders a sense of well being, and undoubtedly some patients experience a placebo response. Some become almost euphoric at their ability to walk unlimited distances again. If at eight weeks they can still not walk a mile, the drug is discontinued. The responders have had variable lengths of treatment. Some have relapsed, and others maintained progress after cessation of the drug (Porter and Hibbert, 1983).

We have found this a useful first line of treatment. The responders avoid a surgical decompression, and the non-responders, although willing to have had a course of injections, may prefer to decline surgery. A return of claudicating symptoms after a previous decompression is no contra-indication for Calcitonin. We have observed no serious side effects, but would withhold the drug from women of the child-bearing age.

The mechanism of response to Calcitonin if not placebo is probably vascular. It is too rapid to be due to remodelling of the bone. Canal measurements using ultrasound have not shown any increase in diameter in sixteen responding patients with neurogenic claudication, nor in three patients whose Paget's paraparesis recovered with Calcitonin (Douglas et al, 1981). Likewise, a response in post-operative patients who have relapsed after a previous decompression, is not likely to be due to bony remodelling. Calcitonin may improve the radicular circulation by selectively reducing the intraosseous blood supply via the branches of the lumbar arteries. This drug does reduce skeletal blood flow (Wooton et al, 1981), and it could stimulate a shunt mechanism providing for a deprived cauda equina. Venous blood drains from the vertebral bodies into Batson's extradural plexus, and if this is likewise reduced, the neural elements will enjoy more space.

If symptoms of claudication are sufficiently severe they are generally relieved by surgical decompression (Verbiest, 1977, Crock, 1981, Parke et al, 1981) (Fig. 14.12). Most patients are immediately impressed with the improved sensation in their legs and are soon walking long distances. Not a few relapse as a laminectomy membrane of fibrous tissue develops over the posterior dura. Their walking distance again becomes reduced. Verbiest recorded that 70 out of 74

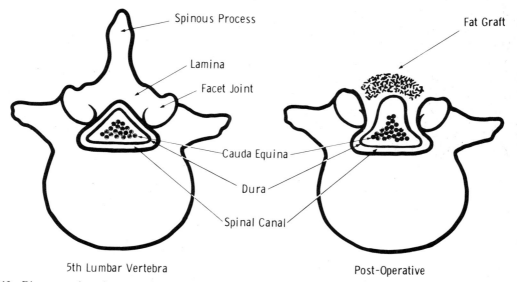

Spinous Process

Lamina

Facet Joint

Fat Graft

Cauda Equina

Dura

Spinal Canal

5th Lumbar Vertebra

Post-Operative

Fig. 14.12 Diagram to show decompression of the cauda equina by excision of the laminae and spinous process and undercutting of the facets. The dura bulges between the facets and is protected from iatrogenic scarring by a free fat graft.

of his patients with neurogenic claudication were relieved by decompression (1977) and this probably depends on careful patient selection and adequate decompression. Russin and Sheldon (1976) and Lassale et al (1984) likewise recorded excellent long term follow up results with decompression for stenotic symptoms but back pain is the most common persisting problem (Getty, 1980). Advanced age is no contra-indication to decompression; it will often improve the quality of life for the elderly (Ami Hood and Weigl, 1983). Some results are less satisfactory and in these it is claimed that decompression was less than adequate, that arachnoiditis spoilt the results, or that longstanding ischaemia of the nerve roots became irreversible. Most operative series have a hard core of failures. A year after decompression, 15 per cent of our patients were completely free of symptoms, 55 per cent were improved, but still had some walking pain, and 30 per cent were no better. We tend to offer surgical decompression, therefore, to those patients who have not responded to Calcitonin, and to those most severely disabled. About half of the patients not responding to Calcitonin will prefer to accept their walking limitations and live with them, rather than submit to a spinal operation. The rest will accept a surgical remedy. The spinal compression must be adequate (Schatzker and Pennal, 1968, Wiltse et al, 1976). It must extend sufficiently proximal to permit a free flow of cerebrospinal fluid to the distal cauda equina and it must be sufficiently lateral to ensure that there is no occlusion of the nerve roots. It usually involves removing three laminae with the spinous processes, sometimes two, and occasionally four. The results of one or two level decompression for localised segmental stenosis seems to give better long term results than a more extensive three, four or five level decompression for multi level disease (Grabias, 1980). The canal will have been narrow for years prior to the development of symptoms and although there may be stenosis at multiple levels, the symptomatic pathology is probably localised. The operative dilemma is to ensure that this critical segment is effectively decompressed. One tends to rely upon an intra-operative clinical impression that the tight dura and roots are given adequate space, and on the grounds of safety one may at times be more radical than is necessary. Somato sensory evoked potentials may have a place as an intra operative diagnostic aid to the extent of decompression (Kiem et al, 1984).

If there is a degenerative spondylolisthesis it is essential not to increase the instability of that segment unnecessarily (Lin, 1982) but forward post operative displacement is unusual even with wide decompression and even with a pre-existing degenerative spondylolisthesis (Grabias 1980 and Shenkin and Hash, 1976). The integrity of the apophyseal joints is not unduly disturbed though the medial third of the joint must often be removed and the facet undercut. It is necessary to perform a decompression wide enough to ensure a completely free dura (Wiltse et al, 1976) but not too wide to produce either instability or such a shallow spinal gutter that a laminectomy membrane will soon compress the dura to a ribbon.

Provided there is no degenerative spondylolisthesis, it is legitimate to sacrifice the major part of the apophyseal joint on one side in order to obtain satisfactory decompression, and not jeopardise stability.

A fat graft applied over the decompressed dura reduces the risk of post-operative fibrous compression. To ensure that the fat survives and is revascularised it is applied as thin postage stamp sized grafts rather than one large cube of fat. This is obtained from the sub cutaneous layer at the operation site, but in thin men it may have to be dissected from a separate buttock incision. One should obliterate 'dead space' and secure haemostasis.

Patients are pleased to be mobilised early, in fact it is difficult to restrain them. They find their own limitations and many remain highly satisfied.

REFERENCES

Ami Hood S, Weigl K 1983 Lumbar spinal stenosis: surgical intervention for the older person. Israel Journal of Medical Sciences 19: 169–171

Bergmark 1950 Intermittent spinal claudication. Acta Med Scand 246 (Suppl): 30

Bestawros O A, Vreeland O H, Golman M L 1979 Epidural venography in the diagnosis of lumbar spinal stenosis. Radiology 131: 423–426

Birkensfield R, Kasdon D L 1978 Congenital lumbar ridge causing spinal claudication in adolescents. Journal of Neurosurgery 49: 441–444

Black K A, McCormick C, Owen E T, Vaughan R 1982 Spinal stenosis: a review of 23 cases. Journal of Rheumatology 9: 573–578

Blau J N, Logue V 1978 The natural history of intermittent claudication of the cauda equina. Brain 101: 211–222

Blau J N, Rushworth G 1958 Observations of blood vessels of the spinal cord and their responses to motor activity. Brain 81: 354–363

Bowen V, Shannan R, Kirkcaldy-Willis W H 1978 Lumbar spinal stenosis. Child's Brain 4: 257–277

Buchthal F 1949 Problems of the pathologic physiology of poliomyelitis. American Journal of Medicine 6: 587–591

Brish A, Lerner M B, Braham J 1964 Intermittent claudication from compression of the cauda equina by a narrowed spinal canal. Journal of Neurosurgery 21: 207–211

Charcot J M C 1858 Sur la claudication intermittente observee dans un cas d'obliteration complete de l'une des arteres iliaques primitives. Comptes Rendu Soc Biol 10: 225–238

Critchley E M R 1982 Lumbar spinal stenosis. British Medical Journal 284: 1588–1589

Crock H V 1981 Normal and pathological anatomy of the lumbar spinal nerve root canals. Journal of Bone and Joint Surgery 63–B: 487–490

DeJerine J 1911 La claudication intermittente de la molle epiniere. Press Med 19: 981

Domminisse G F 1975 Morphological aspects of the lumbar spine and lumbo sacral region. Orthopaedic Clinics of North America 6: 163–175

Douglas D L, Duckworth T, Kanis J A, Jefferson A A, Martin T J, Russell R G G 1981 Spinal cord dysfunction in Paget's disease of bone: has medical treatment a vascular basis? Journal of Bone and Joint Surgery 63–B: 495–503

Dyck P, Doyle J B 1977 'Bicycle test' of van Gelderen in diagnosis of intermittent cauda equina compression syndrome. Journal of Neurosurgery 46: 667–670

Dyck P 1979 The Stoop-test in lumbar entrapment radiculography. Spine 4: 89–92

Ehni G 1969 Significance of the small lumbar spinal canal cauda equina compression syndromes due to spondylosis. Journal of Neurosurgery 31: 490–494

Gathier J C 1959 A case of absolute stenosis of the lumbar vertebral canal in adults. Acta Neuro chir (Wein) 7: 344–349

Getty C J M 1980 Lumbar spinal stenosis: the clinical spectrum and the results of operation. Journal of Bone and Joint Surgery 62–B: 481–485

Grabias S 1980 Current concepts review the treatment of spinal stenosis. Journal of Bone and Joint Surgery 62–A: 308–313

Herzberg L, Bayliss E 1980 Spinal cord syndrome due to non-compression Paget's disease of bone. Lancet ii: 13–15

Jayson M I V, Nelson M A 1979 Spinal stenosis and low back pain. Rheumatic Diseases 70: Arthritis and Rheumatism Council

Johansson J E, Barrington T W, Ameli M 1982 Combined vascular and neurogenic claudication. Spine 7: 150–158

Kiem H A, Hajdu M, Gonzales E, Brand L and Balasubhramanian 1984 Somatosensory evoked potentials as a diagnostic aid in the diagnosis and intra-operative management of spinal stenosis. Presented to the International Society for the study of the Lumbar Spine, Montreal

Lamberton A J, Bannister R, Withrington R, Seifert M H, Eastcott H H G 1983 Claudication of the sciatic nerve. British Medical Journal 286: 1785–1786

Larson S J, Milwaukee W I 1983 Somatosensory evoked potentials in lumbar stenosis. Surgery Gynaecology and Obstetrics 157: 191–196

Lassale B, De Burge A and Benoist M 1984 Long term results of surgical treatment of lumbar stenosis. Presented to the International Society for the study of the Lumbar Spine, Montreal

Lin P M 1982 Internal decompression for multiple levels of lumbar spinal stenosis: a technical note. Neurosurgery 11: 546–549

Magnaes B 1982 Clinical recording of pressure on the spinal cord and cauda equina. Journal of Neurosurgery 57: 57–63

Park W W, Gammell K, Rothman R H 1981 Arterial vascularisation of the cauda equina. Journal of Bone and Joint Surgery 63–A: 53–6

Porter R W 1982 Relief work, spinal decompression. Nursing Mirror 42–44

Porter R W, Hibbert C 1983 Calcitonin treatment for neurogenic claudication. Spine 8: 585–592

Ravichandran G 1981 Spinal cord function in Paget's disease of spine. Paraplegia 19: 7–11

Reichert F L, Ryland D A, Bruck E L 1934 Arteriosclerosis of the lumbar segmental arteries producing ischaemia of the spinal cord and consequent claudication of the thighs. American Journal of Medical Science 187: 794–806

Rosenberg N J 1976 Degenerative spondylolisthesis. Clinical Orthopaedics and Related Research 117: 112–120

Russin L A, Sheldon J 1976 Spinal stenosis. Report of series and long term follow up. Clinical Orthopaedics 115: 101–103

Salibi B S 1976 Neurogenic claudication and stenosis of the lumbar spinal canal. Surgical Neurology 5: 269–272

Schatzker J, Pennal G F 1968 Spinal stenosis, a cause of cauda equina compression. Journal of Bone and Joint Surgery 50–B: 606–618

Shenkin H A, Hash C J 1976 A new approach to the surgical treatment of lumbar spondylosis. Journal of Neurosurgery 44: 148–155

Simkin P A 1982 Simian stance: a sign of spinal stenosis. The Lancet 652–653

van Gelderen C 1948 Ein orthotisches (lodotisches) Kaudasyndrom. Acta Psychatr Neurol 23: 57–68

van Gelderen V 1958 Ein orthotisches (lordotisches) kauda syndrom. Acta Psychatr Neurol Scand 23: 57

Venner R M, Crock H V 1981 Clinical studies of isolated disc resorption in the lumbar spine. Journal of Bone and Joint Surgery 63–B: 491–494

Verbiest H 1954 A radicular syndrome from developmental narrowing of the lumbar vertebral canal. Journal of Bone and Joint Surgery 36–B: 230

Verbiest H 1977 Results of surgical treatment of idiopathic developmental stenosis of the lumbar vertebral canal. A review of twenty seven years' experience. Journal of Bone and Joint Surgery 59–B: 181–188

Walpin L A, Singer F R 1979 Paget's disease, reversal of severe paraparesis with calcitonin. Spine 4: 213–219

Weisz G M 1983 Lumbar spinal canal stenosis in Paget's disease. Spine 8: 192–198

Williams R W 1975 The narrow lumbar spinal canal. Australasian Radiology 19: 356–360

Wilson C B, Brill F R 1977 Spinal stenosis. The narrow lumbar spinal canal syndrome. Clinical Orthopaedics 122: 244–248

Wiltse L L, Newman P H, Macnab I 1976 Classification of spondylolysis and spondylolisthesis. Clinical Orthopaedics and Related Research 117: 23–29

Wooton R, Tellez M, Green J R, Reeve J 1981 Skeletal blood flow in Paget's disease of bone. Metabolic Bone Disease and Related Research 4 & 5: 263–270

15

Segmental instability — biomechanical definition, symptoms, signs, radiological features and management

There is at present no general agreement on the definition, the pathology or the clinical manifestation of lumbar instability. It is accepted, however, that the spine should in health move as a unit, like a flexible rod with a defined arc of rotation, but because of its segmental anatomy, it is possible for some unnatural movement to take place at one or more intervertebral levels.

BIOMECHANICAL DEFINITION

A system may be in stable, neutral or unstable equilibrium (Fig. 15.1). A stable equilibrium occurs in the spine when deformation is accompanied by full recovery. A neutral equilibrium develops when there is segmental displacement of the spine in any of the three axes of rotation, forwards or backwards, (spondylolisthesis or retro-spondylolisthesis) sideways such as may accompany a scoliosis, or rotational instability (Farfan, 1973). There is displacement but stability, a neutral equilibrium, if segmental movements of the displacement are within the limits of normal restraint.

An unstable spine occurs when there is deformation beyond the limits of normal restraint. In practice it returns again to the pre-deformation state. It can occur when a located spine deforms; alternatively a displaced spine, initially in a state of neutral equilibrium, can become unstable as it deforms beyond the limit of normal restraint, and in practice it too returns to the pre-deformation state, though still displaced.

SYMPTOMS OF INSTABILITY

A displaced vertebra in neutral equilibrium may produce no symptoms. In fact, gross displacement in any of the three planes may be present for many years before symptoms develop, if they occur at all. Symptoms are more likely to occur from postural changes in the presence of vertebral displacement because of the pre-existing neurological displacement.

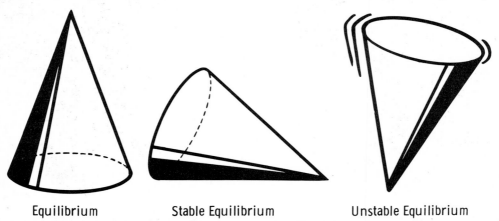

Equilibrium   Stable Equilibrium   Unstable Equilibrium

Fig. 15.1 Diagram to demonstrate systems which are in stable equilibrium (the upright cone will return to the same position if disturbed); neutral equilibrium (the cone on its side will stay in the displaced position); and unstable equilibrium (the cone on end will move into a new position of equilibrium) (Pope and Panjabi 1985).

Thus, dural pain, root pain and neurogenic claudication are all more probable when there is some vertebral displacement in any of the three planes, especially with an intact neural arch, but provided the postural change is not beyond the bound of normal restraint, these symptoms should not be considered symptoms of instability, only associated symptoms.

It is the symptoms that are associated with excessive unnatural movement, that should rightly be considered symptoms of instability. That is, when a located or displaced vertebra deforms beyond the normal restraint and yet returns again to the pre-deformed state. These symptoms are of two types;

1. *Symptoms of fatigue in the structures which restrain shear.* The posterior bony elements of the vertebral arch, with coronally orientated lower lumbar apophyseal joints are the major restraining structures. When these fail, either by deficiency in the pars interarticularis, or by disorganisation of the apophyseal joints, the ligamentous and muscular structures are liable to fatigue (Ferguson, 1933, Wyke, 1980). This probably results in backache with or without referred pain round the pelvis or into the posterior thighs. It is aggravated by walking far, especially shopping, which involves stopping and starting, and carrying. Neither can these patients stand for long. They lie down for relief, when the pain settles completely. It is aggravated by obesity and pregnancy.

2. *Symptoms of momentary subluxation.* The pain source may be in the apophyseal joints, in the ligamentous structures or in the dura. It is experienced as the deformed spine returns to the pre-deformation position, in any one of the three axes of rotation. Typically, a patient says that they have discomfort when rising from the stooped position, or pain when getting out of a low chair, (Fig. 15.2). They state that when getting up from sitting they

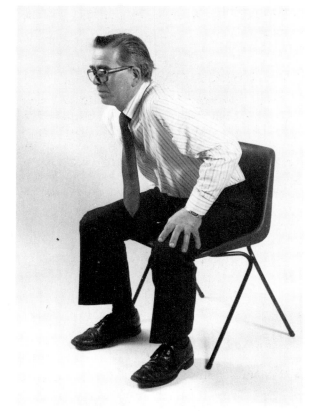

Fig. 15.2A When rising from a chair a patient with instability symptoms will flex the hips to move the centre of gravity forwards.

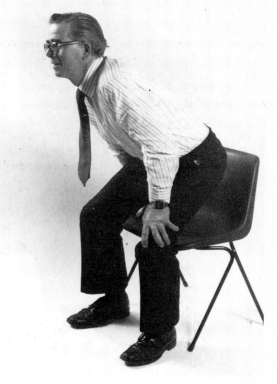

Fig. 15.2B He will then use his hands for support when standing upright. He will sometimes move to the front edge of the chair to place his centre of gravity over his feet prior to rising.

have to support themselves by taking their weight with their hands on the arms of a chair.

The two types of instability symptoms, fatigue and momentary subluxation, may occur independently, or co-exist.

SIGNS OF INSTABILITY

The paraspinal muscles may be hypertrophied, though this is certainly a very subjective sign (Fig. 8.5, page 52). Good paraspinal muscles may be present without instability, and obesity may mask muscle hypertrophy.

The patient with symptoms from an unstable lumbar spine frequently exhibits an exceptionally good range of forward flexion. Many can reach down to their toes with the knees straight, some to put their hands flat on the floor, (combined S.L.R. and spinal flexion). If they are compared as a group, they perform no better than the general population, but they are better than other patients with back pain (Table 16.1, page 134). Most other back pain syndromes restrict forward flexion, probably because the dura and the neural elements are involved as a factor in the symptomatology. Perhaps flexion is unimpaired, because the symptoms of instability are not always related to the contents and space in the vertebral canal.

A patient with symptoms of momentary subluxation will have a classical pattern of spinal motion when standing up again from the stooped position. The normal smooth motion of the spine is broken by a sudden jerky movement, the extension catch. To prevent this, some patients will use their hands to support the spine as they stand up straight from the stooped posture, by 'climbing up their legs' (Fig. 15.3), as also they will rise from a chair.

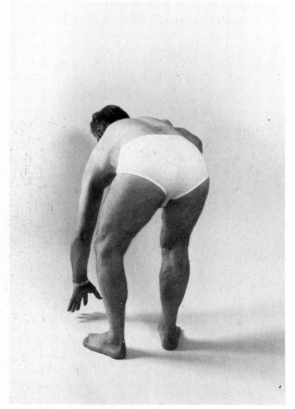

Fig. 15.3A   A patient with instability symptoms often experiences discomfort rising from the stooped position.

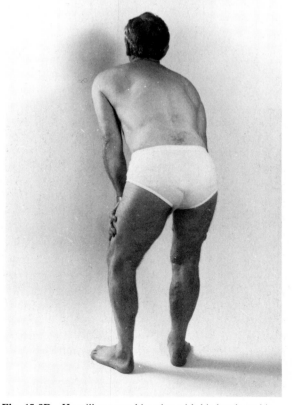

Fig. 15.3B   He will support his spine with his hands on his thighs.

RADIOLOGICAL FEATURES OF INSTABILITY

Instability symptoms are often associated with radiological changes. Herkowitz et al (1983) suggested that more than 2 millimeters of segmental displacement on flexion or extension radiographs is evidence of instability, but any measurement is arbitrary, (Fig. 15.4). Disc space narrowing with traction spurs of the two adjacent vertebrae indicates an unstable segment, (Fig. 13.4, page 106) (Macnab, 1971). A lytic pars is potentially unstable.

There is really no uniform agreement about the value of flexion and extension radiographs, partly because the degree of segmental movement does not correlate with symptoms. Using conventional radiography, Mensor and Duvall (1959) found increased motion at L.4/5 in a similar number of patients with and without back pain. Video radiographs are no more helpful. Steroscopic radiography is producing interesting information about segmental movement, in health and disease, but has yet to be applied to the clinically unstable back (Pearcy et al, 1984). Although the symptoms are not necessarily related to space within the vertebral canal, if space is restricted then unnatural segmental movement can compromise the canal's contents (Fig.

15.5). Other symptoms then coexist with instability, and flexion and exetension views are helpful.

Segmental motion can be assessed in vitro by computor analysis of flexion radiographs of isolated segments, identifying the centrode and recording its change in position and its length. The position and length of the centrode is fairly uniform for non degenerate discs, but degenerative change is associated with erratic movement of the centrode, and an increase in its length. It is not surprising that this is more marked in the mildly degenerate spine than with gross degeneration (Seligmen et al, 1984).

The divorce between biomechanical instability and symptoms results in a clinical dilemma. Gross displacement may be symptomless, and mild instability troublesome. Typical symptoms may not be associated with any abnormal radiological changes at all. Frequently, however, there are radiological features that match the symptoms, and make 'instability' a recognizable back pain syndrome.

TREATMENT OF INSTABILITY

The severity of the symptoms, the degree of disturbance they produce in family and working life, the expectancy of the patient — these will dictate the way in which the problem is managed.

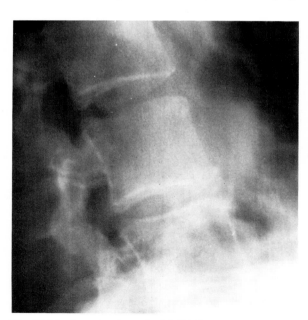

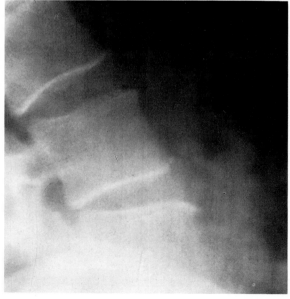

Fig. 15.4A Lateral radiograph of L.3/4 disc space in flexion — small traction spurs.

Fig. 15.4B In extension there is evidence of segmental instability with some posterior displacement of L.3.

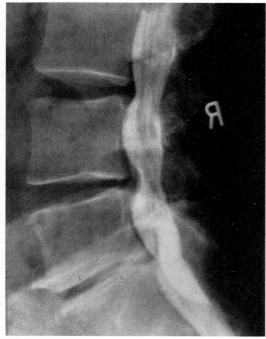

Fig. 15.5A   Lateral radiograph showing posterior dural displacement at L.4/5 in extension.

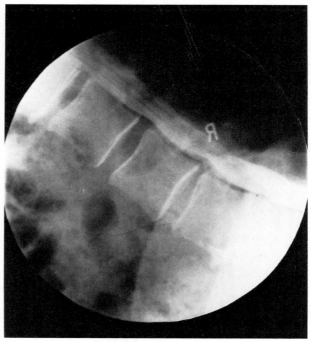

Fig. 15.5B   In flexion the dural bulge is largely corrected.

Symptoms of fatigue which develops after standing, walking about and shopping, may be either a mild intermittent nuisance, or a severe disability. Most patients are seeking a diagnosis, and advice about their future prospects, and ways of making the discomfort manageable. The mechanism of the pain is easily described. Even though they cannot be promised a cure with the passage of time, it is usually possible to say that with care, the symptoms will probably not get worse. If they are obese, it is worth taking weight reduction seriously. Simple advice like using a shopping trolley, not walking further than necessary, using a stick for longer distances, not standing too long, getting a high stool to perch on in the kitchen, these are all ways to reduce the shear forces on the spine. The advice can be reinforced in a 'Back School' situation, reducing the level of apprehension about backache. They are advised to avoid stooping forward more than necessary, and to avoid lifting in the stooped position. They may need to modify their working environment, even change their job if that is practical. The 'Back School' situation is ideal, in order to spend time with the

patient looking at their activities through a normal day. Many will be helped by wearing a lumbo-sacral corset intermittently, say at work or when shopping.

An acute exacerbation of the fatigue pain, with constant ambulant pain in the lower back and perhaps in the thighs can be improved by wearing a plaster jacket for three months. A longer period in plaster, or in a rigid support, is counter-productive.

Apart from the obese woman with degenerative spondylolisthesis, and some patients with isthmic spondylolisthesis, the prognosis can be good. Many a subluxating unstable spine becomes stable as the spine stiffens with the years. Patients learn to avoid the movement that produces pain, and that arc of movement is eventually lost. The fact that instability symptoms generally present in the fifth decade, suggests that time lessens the problem.

Indications for surgery

For a few however this reassurance is inadequate; occasionally the fatigue pain is of such intensity and duration that it interferes with normal life and surgery must be considered. If the segmental level of the pain source can be confidently identified, and if a spinal fusion of that segment can be guaranteed, it should be possible to promise a cure. Surgical failure results from either making the wrong diagnosis, or from not obtaining a satisfactory fusion.

Surgical assessment follows a logical sequence.

— *Is the diagnosis correct?* If the symptoms suggest that the back pain and referred pain originate from an unstable segment, and if this is supported by abnormal signs, further investigations may help. A myelogram is often normal, but a discogram should confirm disc degeneration. An abnormal discogram does not, of course, mean that this is the level of the pain source. Provocative discography simulating the distribution of pain does not guarantee that this is the pain source. One of the main problems about fusing a spine for symptoms of instability, is that even in isthmic spondylolysis, one has presumptive evidence only about the pain source. A policy of random fusion for severe backache will only result in a hard core of failure.

— *Is the disability sufficiently severe, and has it persisted sufficiently long to make surgery worthwhile?* The majority of patients with instability who do not

respond to conservative management have an isthmic spondylolisthesis, and even these, if observed for a period of time, may respond to reducing spinal stess, and a period in plaster.

— *Is there a possibility of exaggeration of the symptoms?* The surgeon is generally persuaded to operate because of the degree and persistence of the patient's symptoms, and therefore objective assessment of the disability is essential. Are there many inappropriate symptoms in addition to the back and referred pain? Are there inappropriate signs? What is the psychological profile? The results of surgery can be less than successful if there is evidence of exaggeration of the symptoms.

— *What is the state of the segment proximal to the proposed fusion segment?* A fusion should not be attempted unless the disc above the proposed fusion can be shown to be normal by discogram. If degenerate, it could be the pain source, and a more distal fusion will only add to the patient's problem, increasing that instability, (Fig. 15.6). The vertebral canal at the proximal end of the proposed fusion should be of adequate dimensions. Even a normal segment proximal to the fusion, could become

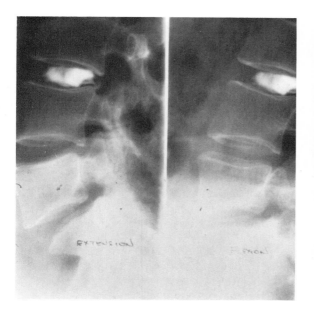

Fig. 15.6A Lateral radiograph of a patient with segmental instability at L.4/5 level showing unnatural movement in extension on the left and flexion on the right. This is the segment above an isthmic spondylolisthesis at L.5/S.1. The L.3/4 discogram shows that this disc is also degenerate.

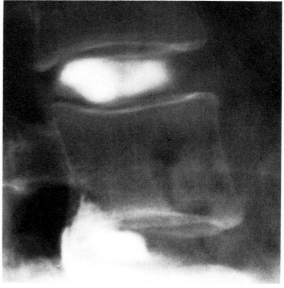

Fig. 15.6B A discogram of the unstable L.4/5 segment shows an annular tear with extravasation posteriorly. A fusion from L.4 to S.1 may be successful but the pathological L.3/4 disc may jeopardise surgical success.

unstable from the added stresses that will be applied to it, and if the canal is already narrow, it could eventually cause stenosis symptoms.

Technique for spinal fusion

Each method has its own advocates.

— *Posterior spinal fusion was developed by Hibbs (1911) and has received several modifications.* After removing the cortex from the posterior neural arch, and the articular cartilage from the apophyseal joints, the area is packed with cancellous bone from the posterior iliac crest. Screws across the apophyseal joints (Boucher, 1959) or dowel grafts provide a measure of internal fixation. A posterior iliac crest 'H' graft held in situ by compression springs, (Attenborough and Reynolds, 1975), provides a secure and effective fusion. The graft does not lift off its bed in flexion, but becomes more firmly apposed by the tightening springs.

— *Postero-lateral and intertransverse fusions are perhaps the most widely practised method of fusion* (Adkins, 1955, Wiltse et al, 1968, Crock 1983) through a muscle splitting exposure three fingers breadths lateral to the mid line. This does allow for a spinal decompression if necessary.

— *A Buck fusion* through the pars interarticularis is useful in lytic spondylolisthesis.

— *An anterior interbody fusion* replacing the intervertebral disc and cartilage end plates has its devotees (Goldner et al, 1971) but it carries its own complications of paralytic ileus, urinary retention, incisional hernia and impotence. There is a place for incorporating anterior and posterior fusion, (O'Brien 1983).

The symptoms of momentary subluxation, discomfort rising from the stooped position or when getting out of a chair, are unpleasant and a nuisance, but are rarely disabling, unless associated with other problems. Most patients fortunately do not need surgery and can be managed satisfactorily with an explanation of the mechanics of the pain, and advice about management and prognosis.

REFERENCES

Adkins E W O 1955 Lumbosacral arthrodes is after laminectomy. Journal of Bone and Joint Surgery 37–B: 208

Attenborough C G, Reynolds M T 1975 Lumbo-sacral fusion with spring fixation. Journal of Bone and Joint Surgery 57–B: 283–288

Boucher H H 1959 A method of spinal fusion. Journal of Bone and Joint Surgery 41–B: 248

Crock H V 1983 Practice of spinal surgery. Springer-Verlag Wein New York.

Farfan H G 1973 The mechanical disorders of the lower back. Philadelphia, Lea and Febiger

Ferguson A B 1933 The clinical and roentgenographic interpretation of lumbo-sacral anomalies. Radiology 22: 548–558

Goldner J L, Urbaniak J R, McCollum D E 1971 Anterior disc excision and interbody spinal fusion for chronic low back pain. Orthopaedic Clinics of North America 2: 543

Herkowitz H N, Romeyn R L, Rothman R H 1983 The indications for metrizamide myelography. Journal of Bone and Joint Surgery 65–A: 1144–1149

Hibbs R A 1911 An operation for progressive spinal deformities. New York Medical Journal 93: 1013

Macnab I 1971 The traction spur. Journal of Bone and Joint Surgery 53–A: 663–670

Mensor M C, Duvall G 1959 Absence of motion at the fourth and fifth lumbar interspaces in patients with and without low back pain. Journal of Bone and Joint Surgery 41–A: 1047–1054

O'Brien J P 1983 The role of fusion for chronic low back pain. The Orthopaedic Clinics of North America 14: 639–647

Pearcy M, Portek I, Shepherd J E 1984 Three dimensional x-ray analysis of normal movement in the lumbar spine. Spine (in press)

Pope N H, Panjabi M 1985 Biomechanical definitions of spinal instability. Spine 10: 255–256

Seligmen J V, Gertzbein S D and Tile M 1984 Computor analysis of spinal segment motion in degenerative disc disease with and without axial loading. Presented to the International Society for the study of the Lumbar Spine, Montreal

Wiltse L L, Bateman J G, Hutchinson R H, Nelson W E 1968. The paraspina; sacrospinalis splitting approach to the lumbar spine. Journal of Bone and Joint Surgery 50–A: 919–926

Wyke B D 1980 The neurology of low back pain. Chapter 11 in The Lumbar Spine and Back Pain, 2nd edition, p 265–339. Ed. by M I V Jayson, Pitman Medical, London

16

Lysis of the pars interarticularis — pathology, identification of the defect, clinical significance and management

PATHOLOGY

Lysis of the pars interarticularis continues to interest clinicians treating back pain, because it is assumed that such an obvious anatomical anomaly must have symptomatic significance. It is, however, a relatively common condition, frequently symptomless, with a variable incidence amongst selected groups. Roche and Rowe (1951) carried out a large study of white skeletons, and found an overall incidence of bilateral lysis in 4.2 per cent of 2,300 skeletons, there being a male to female ratio of almost three to one. Studies in vivo have shown a greater incidence in selected athletic groups, from 5 per cent to 21 per cent (Kono et al, 1975, Troup, 1975, Jackson et al, 1976, Murray-Leslie et al, 1977, Bird et al, 1980 and Hitoshi, 1980).

It is generally accepted that the lysis has a traumatic origin, but some individuals may be constitutionally predisposed to develop a defect (Newman, 1963, Farfan, 1973, Fredrickson et al, 1984). The existence of unilateral spondylolysis suggests that not all lytic defects result from trauma, though probably most of them do. The high incidence amongst the Eskimo races led Roche and Rowe (1951) to suspect that it was a congenital condition but they later modified their views (1953) suggesting that certain postures adopted by the Eskimo may generate unacceptable high stresses in the pars interarticularis, causing a stress fracture. Troup (1975) has shown that the shearing forces across the pars are particularly high in forced spinal extension and such repetitive forces in gymnasts and other athletes may account for their high incidence. It could equally be argued however, that an athletic career is often chosen by subjects with lysis because they are in some respects hypermobile. We are equally ignorant about the aietology of

spondylolysis and about the factors responsible for the variable degree of displacement.

Lysis of the pars is more common at L.5 than at L.4 (Fig. 16.1). It occasionally occurs sequentially up the lumbar spine in athletes whose spines are subject to high torque, ie. fast bowlers.

The displacement when it occurs is usually only to a moderate degree but lysis can occur with no vertebral displacement at all (spondylolysis) or the proximal vertebra may be completely dislocated. It is expressed as a percentage of the forward displacement of the posterior margin of the proximal vertebral body, over the antero-posterior diameter of the vertebra below (Fig. 9.2, page 59) (Blackburne and Velikas, 1977, Wiltse and Winter. 1983). The mean displacement of 162 patients attending our clinic with lysis was 17 per cent and only 4 patients had a slip ratio greater than 40 per cent. Gross displacement is usually associated with congenital anomalies of the posterior vertebral arch, a wide spina bifida and attenuation of the pars — 'dysplastic spondylolisthesis'. Wiltse, Newman and Macnab (1976) in their classification, distinguished this from the more common 'isthmic spondylolisthesis', where there is a lytic defect of the pars without dysplasia. Sometimes the difference is more apparent than real, and the two may be but extremes of one condition.

Conditions other than lysis of the pars can result in spondylolisthesis, an acute fracture — 'Traumatic spondylolisthesis', generalised or localised bone pathology — 'Pathological spondylolisthesis' and 'Degenerative spondylolisthesis' (Chapter 18).

The term 'slip' is a misnomer. The degree of displacement has not been shown to suddenly increase with a forward slip. Displacement can be shown to progress gradually during childhood (Fig. 16.2) but after maturity, displacement at least at

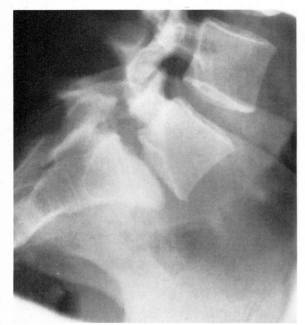

Fig. 16.1A Lateral radiograph of patient with lysis of pars interarticularis at L.5.

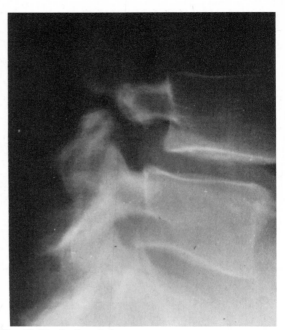

Fig. 16.1B   Lysis at L.4.

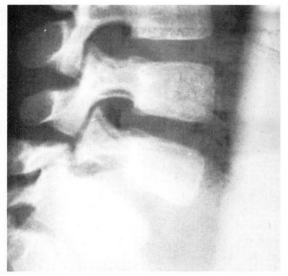

Fig. 16.2A   Lateral radiograph of a 7 year old girl with isthmic spondylolisthesis and a slip ratio of 34 per cent.

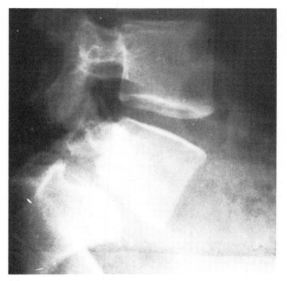

Fig. 16.2B   At 18 years of age the slip ratio had increased to 40 per cent. Most of the displacement has occurred before seven years of age.

L5/S1 does not increase significantly (Fig. 16.3). The displacement should rather be considered a growth phenomenon, with gradual remodelling of the posterior vertebral elements in response to the forces of shear. The degree of displacement that exists at

maturity probably changes little thereafter. This growth concept is supported by the asymmetrical **development of vertebrae with unilateral spondylolysis (Chapter 17, p. 143).**

About one patient in four with a lysis will clearly

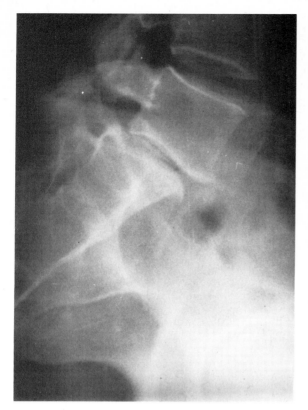

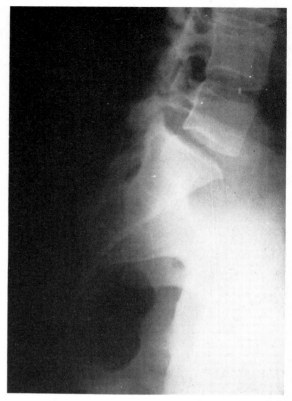

Fig. 16.3A Lateral radiograph of a 63 year old woman with isthmic spondylolisthesis at L.5/S.1 and a slip ratio of 17 per cent.

Fig. 16.3B Radiograph of the same patient at 34 years of age when the slip ratio was 13 per cent.

recollect a childhood injury to the spine. They remember a fall downstairs, from a wall or tree. If such an injury were to damage a pre-existing lytic defect of the pars, and result in instability, the posterior elements would not then be able to adequately restrain the shear forces. Growth remodelling would then allow progressive displacement until maturity. The age at which such an injury occurred would effect the degree of displacement. Hitchcock (1940) has suggested that the hyper-flexion and torsion of a traumatic birth delivery could fracture the pars. He produced neural arch fractures by cadavaric experiments, but this was not supported by the work of Rowe and Roche (1953). If birth injury were a significant factor in the development of a lysis, one would expect spondylolysis to be uncommon in children born by Caesarean section. Only one of our 162 patients with lysis of the pars had been born by Caesarean section,

far less than the 5 per cent section rate in the 1940s. Perhaps birth injury is significant.

Although the aetiology of isthmic spondylolisthesis is unresolved, it is a good working hypothesis to accept that some individuals are pre-disposed to develop a lysis of the pars; that it probably occurs very early in life; that it is usually stable, being adequately supported by soft tissues which restrain the shear forces and prevent forward displacement; that some subjects injure the site of the existing defect causing instability; and the unrestrained shear forces then result in a growth remodelling process with forward displacement of the proximal segment. The degree of that displacement will depend on two factors, the age at which the instability occurs, and the degree with which the soft tissues are able to withstand shear.

Tensile forces develop across the pars from the downward pull of the muscles attached to the spinous processes, and the shear forces across the disc (Stott et al, 1981). These forces are acceptable in an intact pars, and are presumably adequately restrained in many a spondylolytic defect. The intact disc itself is a powerful restrainer of shear. The disc at the level of spondylolisthesis has characteristic histology (Roberts et al 1982). The anterior lip of the first sacral body develops a prominence to match the proximal vertebra, partly resisting displacement. Stability may **become absolute by a spontaneous bony fusion (Fig. 16.4 and Fig. 9.3, page 59).**

Should unacceptable bending movements cause an isthmic defect of the pars to become unstable in infancy, and should the soft tissues prove unstable to restrain shear, there will be a long period of growth available for these forces to elongate the pars and for considerable displacement to occur. Displacement by growth would have less time to develop from a similar injury in later childhood. Wiltse and Jackson (1976) noted that displacement increases most rapidly if spondylolisthesis is detected at the start of the growth spurt.

A defect that remains stable throughout growth

may produce no displacement provided the soft tissues maintain that stability.

The ability of the soft tissues to restrain the forces of shear, will affect the degree of displacement. The greatest displacement occurs in 'dysplastic spondylolisthesis' where hypoplastic posterior vertebral elements are also associated with anomalies of the attachments of multifidus and the lumbar fascia. In 'Isthmic spondylolisthesis' there is a high incidence of spina bifida occulta (Fredrickson et al 1984). 32 per cent of our patients had spina bifida at L.5 or at S.1 but these did not have a greater degree of displacement than those without a spina bifida.

The elastic properties of the spinal ligamentous structures may be a factor in vertebral displacement (Bird et al, 1980). This is difficult to measure, but probably the Leeds Hyperextensiometer (Jobbins et al, 1979) is the most useful index of generalised joint mobility (Fig. 16.5). We found a useful correlation of 0.26 ($p < .05$) between the slip ratio of 162 patients with lysis and the hyperextensiometer measurement of the second left metacarpal.

There is a positive correlation between the lumbo sacral angle and the degree of displacement (Blackburne and Velikas 1977). The lumbo sacral angle is best measured between the L.3/4 and L.5/S.1 disc spaces (Farfan, 1973) and in our series this showed a correlation of 0.39 ($p < .01$) with the degree of displacement. It does not follow that an initial steep angle of inclination is related to the speed of displacement. Rather it is probable that as displacement occurs slowly during growth, the body of L.5 becomes gradually wedged (Porter and Park, 1982), and the lumbo-sacral angle in adult life merely

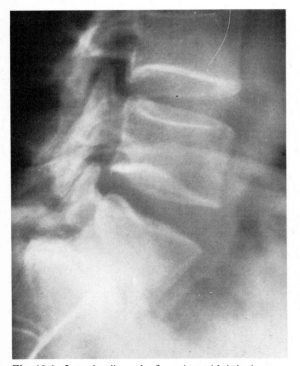

Fig. 16.4 Lateral radiograph of a patient with isthmic spondylolisthesis, elongation of the pars and a 33 per cent slip ratio stabilised by spontaneous fusion.

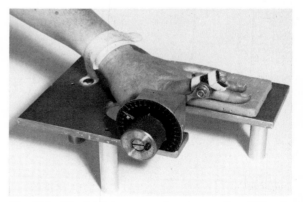

Fig. 16.5 The Leeds hyperextensiometer records mobility of the 2nd left metacarpo phalangeal joint.

reflects the growth change of the vertebral body. However, once established, this increasing angle will produce greater shear forces tending to accelerate the displacement.

Vertebral displacement with elongation of the pars has the advantage of widening the sagittal diameter of the central vertebral canal (Fig. 16.6) and thus protecting the patient to some degree from back pain syndromes that are related to a narrow central canal. The powerful epigenetic influence of the neurological tissue ensures that in the growth remodelling displacement process, the root canal remains adequate for the nerve root.

IDENTIFICATION OF A PARS DEFECT

One may suspect a defect from certain features in the history and examination. The patient who has a long history of pain in the back, referred sometimes to the thighs, perhaps with some childhood injury, would make the clinician think of a lysis, more so if they stated that they were previously of good athletic ability, and that they could feel a 'click' in the back. Some patients will give a history of an industrial accident with some heavy weight falling on the back, or symptoms dating from pregnancy.

Many patients with a lysis seem to be highly flexible. They can bend forwards with straight legs and place the flat of the hands on the floor (Jackson et al, 1976). It is not the lumbar spine that is hypermobile, but this manoeuvre is possible because straight leg raising is so good, often well above ninety degrees. Most patients with back pain are not able to put their hands flat on the floor, because spinal flexion and/or striaght leg raising are limited. Patients with lysis are in distinct contrast to others in the clinic because in spite of their back pain, they are often sufficiently flexible to touch the floor. They are little different to non-back pain subjects, however (Table 16.1).

A careful examiner may be able to detect an unstable lysis by palpating the lower lumbar spinous processes first in the neutral position, and then in maximum rotation. The patient lies on their side, and a finger tip is placed on the lower three spinous processes. The patient is then rotated and in an intact spine the processes move in step. The process of L.5 will not move with L.4 if there is an unstable lysis at L.5 (Fig. 8.6, page 53).

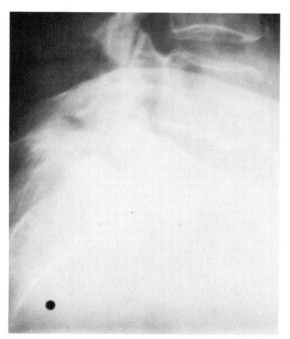

Fig. 16.6A Lateral radiograph of patient with isthmic spondylolisthesis and 40 per cent slip ratio.

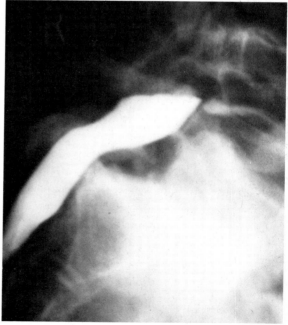

Fig. 16.6B A myelogram shows that the displacement has produced a capacious vertebral canal.

Table 16.1 Ability of patients with isthmic and degenerative spondylolisthesis to flex forwards with straight knees, compared with other patients and volunteer subjects

	Isthmic Spondylolisthesis (n − 98)	Degenerative Spondylolisthesis (n − 53)	Patients with back pain but no spondylolisthesis (n − 115)	Volunteer subjects without back pain (n − 61)
Able to place flat of hands on floor	18%	21%	9%	23%
Able to touch floor with finger tips	35%	36%	22%	62%
Unable to touch the floor	47%	43%	69%	15%

The mid-line hollow created by a forward displaced vertebra will be obvious, both to inspection (Fig. 16.7) and palpation of the back.

A displaced vertebra can usually be recognised by ultrasound examination (Fig. 16.8) when by virtue of the forward rotational element of the displacement, it is more obviously out of line than in radiographic examination.

If the lysis is not obvious on a lateral radiograph, oblique 45 degree projections will usually demonstrate the defect, with the typical 'scottie dog collar effect' (Fig. 9.4, page 60). This may be enhanced by cranial projections (Porter and Park, 1982, Lisbon and Bloom, 1983).

Increased vascularity of the pars interarticularis can be demonstrated by scintigraphy after spinal trauma. It is not possible to say whether this is evidence of a stress fracture in an inherently weakened pars, or disruption of a pre-existing pars defect.

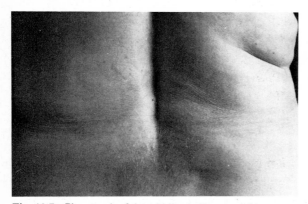

Fig. 16.7 Photograph of the mid line hollow created by a spondylolisthesis.

CLINICAL SIGNIFICANCE

We are tempted to assume that lysis of the pars is in some way the cause of a patient's backache because it is such an obvious anomaly, but both backache and lysis are common, and they may at times be unrelated. Studies of the gymnast's spine in spite of the many series being dissimilar in age, sex and nationality, show two things in common; spondylolysis and spondylolisthesis is common (5–21 per cent); and many of the subjects with a defect have no symptoms.

The lysis was symptomless in 33 per cent of Bird's series (1980), and in 45 per cent of Jackson's (1976). In Hitoshi's series (1980), 76 per cent of subjects with lysis were symptomless, there being no significant difference in back pain incidence between those athletes with lysis and those without. Semon and Spengler (1981) reached the same conclusion, finding 27 per cent of 506 college football players had back pain, but only 2.4 per cent had pain and a spondylolisthesis. In the short term, the lysis did not appear to have clinical significance. What then is the relevance of lysis of the pars in a patient complaining of back pain?

1. Back and referred pain

This is the most common problem for a patient with lysis of the pars interarticularis (Table 16.2). One in three attending hospital with a defect will have pain across the back and round the pelvis into the buttocks, and when on their feet for long it will affect the thighs and even the upper calves. It has the characteristics of the fatigue pain of instability, being worse standing, walking far, and especially when

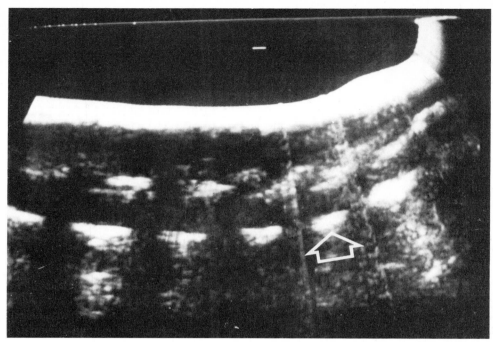

Fig. 16.8   Ultrasound B-scan of 5 lumbar vertebrae and the sacrum showing forward displacement of the body of L.5 and a wide vertebral canal.

Table 16.2   Symptoms associated with 131 patients attending with isthmic spondylolysis or spondylolisthesis

	Percentage of 131 patients with lysis of the pars	Percentage of 2229 patients without lysis of the pars	Significance
Symptomatic disc lesion	1.5	8.7	(p<0.01)
Root entrapment syndrome	16.0	14.1	Not significant
Back and/or referred pain	32.8	18.2	(p<0.001)

shopping. It is relieved lying down. They may add an interesting symptom, that they hear or feel a 'click' in the lower back.

There is often a long history with intermittent pain from childhood, and one in four can remember some violent accident in early life. Others may have a more recent history of an industrial accident when a weight fell on their back. One woman out of five complaining of these symptoms attributes the onset of pain to pregnancy, an observation which is three times more common for women with defects than for other women with back pain (Table 16.3).

They can usually reach well forwards and touch the floor, even with the flat of the hands, and this is accompanied by excellent straight leg raising. An extension catch of subluxating instability is rare. Spinal extension is reduced. There are no abnormal neurological signs.

Investigations are generally unhelpful, radiographs showing no more than a lytic defect and perhaps an olisthesis. The displaced vertebra can be demonstrated by ultrasound, but the vertebral canal measurements are not dissimilar from those of the general population (Table 11.2, page 88).

2. Lower lumbar disc symptoms

It is unusual to encounter a symptomatic disc lesion in a patient with lysis of the pars interarticularis. That is not to say that these patients do not have disc

Table 16.3 Comparison between women with isthmic spondylolisthesis and those without who attributed onset of low back pain to pregnancy

	Percentage who attributed onset of back pain to pregnancy
49 women with lytic defects	20.4%
913 women without lytic defect	6.6%

pathology. In fact, the disc above the vertebra with the lysis is often degenerate (Farfan, 1973) (Fig. 16.9), but the adequate space in the central canal protects the cauda equina. The canal at L.5 is usually dome-shaped in the presence of lysis rather than trefoil (Fig. 16.10) which in itself will ensure that the emerging roots have ample space, even with a disc prolapse. Olisthesis, leaving behind the lamina of L.5 will also increase the mid sagittal diameter of the central canal, ensuring that the roots are compromised neither at L.4/5 nor at L.5/S.1

Classical disc symptoms are therefore unusual with lysis of the pars. A gravity induced list, almost pathognomonic of disc prolapse, is rarely seen in spondylolisthesis. Only 1.5 per cent of our patients with lysis fulfilled McCulloch's criteria for disc

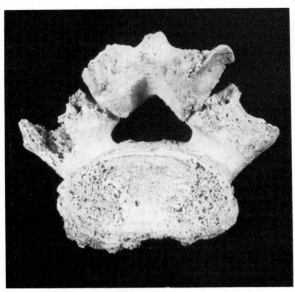

Fig. 16.10A Specimen of 5th lumbar vertebra with bilateral lysis of the pars interarticularis showing adequate vertebral canal even when the neural arch rests on the pedicles. In vivo the separation caused by the defect would further widen the canal.

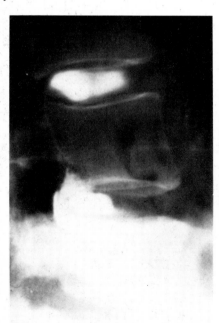

Fig. 16.9 Lateral radiograph of patient with isthmic spondylolisthesis at L.5/S.1 with a degenerate disc at L.4/5 demonstrated by discogram. Symptoms of disc protrusion were avoided by an adequate vertebral canal.

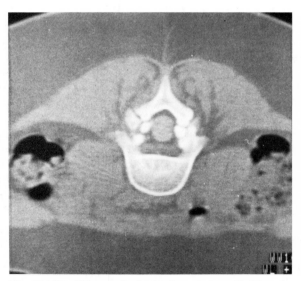

Fig. 16.10B CT scan of a 5th lumbar vertebra with bilateral isthmic defects of the pars interarticularis showing a deep dome shaped central canal.

symptoms (Table 16.2), compared with 8.7 per cent of other back pain patients. There may be many more patients with lysis who have dural pain from a disc prolapse, or who have minimal root signs, but disabling symptoms are rare.

3. Root entrapment syndrome

This occurs with the same frequency in patients with lysis as in other patients. The root is affected sometimes by degenerative changes and by associated soft tissue reaction at the margins of the defect. The dynamic effect of instability may add to the problem by irritating the root in the root canal. A ridge of disc at L.4/5 from a displaced L.5 vertebra can affect the L.5 or S.1 root in the central canal giving root entrapment symptoms. The same root pain may be due to entrapment between the long transverse process of L.5 and the alar of the sacrum, when displacement approaches 40 per cent — the 'far out syndrome' (Wiltse 1982). In spite of gross degenerative change, however, it is surprising that the roots are so often spared (Fig. 16.11).

4. Claudication pain

Many types of spinal pathology can give rise to painful legs when walking (chapter 14), but with a spondylolysis or spondylolisthesis, true neurogenic claudication is uncommon because the canal is so wide. It occasionally results from an unrelated proximal stenotic lesion. Many patients with lysis do have discomfort in the legs which increases with walking and limits the walking distance but it is probably fatigue instability with referred pain into the legs.

5. Spondylolisthesis crisis

The adolescent who has marked displacement of L.5 on S.1 may develop fairly sudden severe symptoms in the back and legs. The crisis is probably due to a relatively acute increase in the forces of shear at S.1. The marked degree of displacement is associated both with wedging of the body of L.5 and increased lumbo-sacral angle, and with the increased weight associated with a growth spurt, instability at the lysis becomes a problem. The vertebral canal which is widened in spondylolisthesis can be distorted by the relatively sudden accelerating displacement. The neural contents have not been able to keep pace with the bony changes, and unnatural movement at the lysis is the final insult to the cauda equina. There is pain in the back and legs, with restricted movements of the spine, spasm, and restricted straight leg raising.

Is the defect of any significance at all?

In a series of 2360 patients attending a back pain clinic, we recorded 5.6 per cent of patients with bilateral lysis of the pars, which is probably no greater than the incidence of the defect in the general population. It could be reasonably suggested that the demonstration of lysis is an incidental finding, unrelated to the cause of back pain. Two facts, however, indicate that the defect can be clinically significant. The first is the considerable difference in the incidence of two back pain syndromes (the symptomatic disc lesion, and back and referred pain) in patients with and without a lysis (Table 16.2). The second observation is that proportionally more women than men who have a lytic defect attend the hospital with back pain. Roche and Rowe (1951) recorded a spondylolisthesis sex ratio of three men to one woman. If this were correct for our population, we have twice as many women attending with lysis than would be expected (a sex ratio of 1.7 to 1).

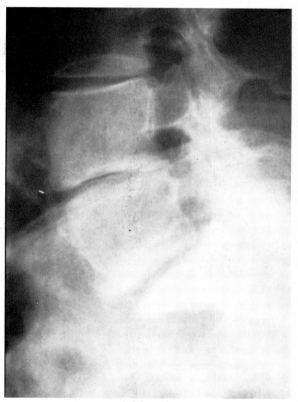

Fig. 16.11 Lateral radiograph of a 74 year old woman with isthmic spondylolisthesis at L.5/S.1 and evidence of disc degeneration at L.4/5. She gave a history of back pain 40 years previously but had no current back or root pain.

Perhaps the effects of pregnancy is important in initiating instability symptoms.

MANAGEMENT OF BACK PAIN AND SPONDYLOLISTHESIS

A spondylolisthesis which is recognised in early life, should not give rise to undue concern. Pain of course can be severe, and ulitmately require surgical treatment, but in general patients with a spondylolysis or spondylolisthesis manage as well as patients without a defect. They are no more likely to visit the hospital with back pain than the rest of the population.

They are more likely than the rest of us to develop back and referred pain, but this is often a manageable problem, and they are better protected against the disabling symptoms of the acute disc lesion.

It would probably be wise for a young man with a known lysis to avoid those occupations where there is a risk of injury from falling weights, but in other respects he is probably a better risk in manual work than others.

A young woman with a known lysis should receive precautionary advice in pregnancy. Here she is at risk of developing instability. She should not be overweight, and should avoid unnecessary lifting and carrying. Frequent periods of rest are advisable, especially in the third trimester. She should be doubly cautious not to fall, and postural advice about pelvic rotation reducing the lumbo-sacral angle, may be useful (Maring-Klug, 1982). Unfortunately, many women progress through pregnancy oblivious of a hidden spondylolisthesis, only to learn of the lesion after subsequent radiography. An earlier diagnosis is possible, if the ultrasonographer performing the first foetal scan will look at every mother's spine for a displaced vertebra.

It is important to spend time describing to a patient what is meant by a spondylolisthesis or they will imagine a slipping vertebra which will eventually dislocate altogether. A few words to explain that the displacement has been present from early life and that it will not materially alter can allay many fears. Each syndrome is then treated on its own merits.

The common problem of pain in the back referred to the thighs is usually managed satisfactorily by an understanding of the instability fatigue pain mechanism and advice about limiting the mechanical stress on the spine. The load carried, its duration and the strength of the spine, are topics for discussion. How can they reduce the amount and frequency of lifting and carrying? Can they improve on their fitness? Are they too heavy? Here is the role of the 'back school'. A good car seat makes a difference, and for those over middle age, there is a place for a lumbo-sacral corset. If there has been a sudden increase in symptoms it is useful to support the spine in a plaster jacket for three months. Most patients with back and referred pain can be effectively managed by conservative means, and although they will probably never be entirely free of symptoms, they can usually cope with the problem. It is the few who cannot adjust that may need surgery. With careful assessment, and a sound fusion (page 128) these are amongst the most grateful of patients (Attenborough and Reynolds, 1975), especially the younger patients with instability type pain (Haraldsson and Willner, 1983).

There is no general agreement about the management of the young athlete with acute low back pain, who has a demonstrable pars defect and a positive scintiscan. If this represents a stress fracture, immobilisation may allow bony union. Some would advocate a plaster spica for three months. The 'hot-spot' may only indicate that a pre-existing lysis has become unstable, and immobilisation is then likely to be unproductive. Some would recommend simply withdrawal from sporting activities. The need for surgical fusion is open to debate, but if symptoms persist which affect an athletic career, it is certainly worthwhile.

A patient with classical disc symptoms may have a lytic defect of the pars which is incidental to the back pain problem. Admittedly these disc symptoms are rare in the presence of a lysis, but the defect may be stable and symptomless, and a protruding disc proximal to the lysis responsible for the root lesion. Management is no different from that offered to other patients with a disc lesion.

Root entrapment occurs in the presence of a lysis, with much the same frequency as in patients without a lysis. The defect, however, is usually a factor in the causation of the symptoms, either from degenerative changes around the lysis of from more proximal or distal involvement. Conservative management for root entrapment is the same as for patients without a defect, though an epidural injection is not likely to influence the 'far out syndrome'. Those few patients requiring surgical help require both adequate decompression of the nerve root and a fusion. Results are not particularly encouraging with a fusion alone (Haraldsson and Willner, 1983). Adequate exposure of L.5 and S.1 is imperative because either root can be responsible for the symptoms at several possible sites, L.5 at the region of the lysis, or from L.4/5 disc level in the central canal, and S.1 from involvement under the cranial lip of the first sacral lamina. If the lesion is in the root canal, then instability forms part of the pathological process and a fusion is necessary. It is also worth while if backache accompanies the root pain. A lateral fusion is the procedure of choice when performing a synchronous decompression.

When the major complaint is painful legs walking, with restricted walking distance, a careful assessment is necessary to find the cause. It is unlikely to be neurogenic claudication because lysis and any displacement tends to widen the vertebral canal. More often the walking pain is instability pain

referred into the thighs, and it is usually managed by conservative means, reducing weight, strengthening the back, and living within the limitations of pain. Only when this is not possible is surgery considered. A fusion will help, provided the canal is wide enough and the proximal discs intact.

Occasionally there is need to fuse an adolescent spine with a spondylolisthesis crisis. A good fusion will relieve the symptoms, and most surgeons would fuse the spine in situ. McPhee and O'Brien (1979) recommends reduction of a severely displaced adolescent spondylolisthesis prior to fusion, to improve the cosmetic appearance.

Johnson and Kirwan (1983) however, reviewed the long term results of fusion in situ for severe spondylolisthesis, and most had excellent ratings twenty years after surgery.

Fortunately, although spondylolysis affects about five per cent of the population, the majority have no symptoms at all, and those who do can be managed without major surgery.

REFERENCES

Attenborough C G, Reynolds M T 1975 Lumbo-sacral fusion with spring fixation. Journal of Bone and Joint Surgery 57-B: 283–288

Bird H A, Eastmond C J, Hudson A, Wright V 1980 Is generalised joint laxity a factor in spondylolisthesis? Scandinavian Journal of Rheumatology 9: 203–205

Blackburne J S, Velikas E P 1977 Spondylolisthesis in children and adolescents. Journal of Bone and Joint Surgery 59-B: 490–494

Farfan H F 1973 The mechanical disorders of the lower back. Philadelphia, Lea and Febiger

Fredrickson B E, Baker D, McHolick W J, Yuan H A, Lubicky J P 1984 The natural history of spondylolysis and spondylolisthesis. Journal of Bone and Joint Surgery 66–A: 699–707

Haraldsson S, Willner S 1983 A comparative study of spondylolisthesis in operations on adolescents and adults. Arch Orthop Trauma Surg 101: 101–105

Hitchcock H H 1940 Spondylolisthesis Journal of Bone and Joint Surgery 22: 1–16

Hitoshi Hoshina 1980 Spondylolysis in athletes. Physician Sports Medicine 8: 75–79

Jackson D W, Wiltse L L, Cirincone R J 1976 Spondylolysis in the female gymnast. Clinical Orthopaedics 117: 68–73

Jobbins B, Bird H A, Wright V 1979 A joint hyperextensiometer for the quantification of joint laxity. Engineering in Medicine 8: 103–105

Johnston J R, Kirwan E O'G 1983 The long term results of fusion in situ for severe spondylolisthesis. Journal of Bone and Joint Surgery 65–B: 43–46

Kono S, Hayashi N, Kashahara G, Akimoto T, Keneko F, Sugiura Y, Harada A 1975 A study of the aetiology of spondylolysis with reference to athletic activities. Journal of Japanese Orthopaedic Association 49: 125–131

Libson E, Bloom R A 1983 Anteroposterior angulated view: a new radiographic technique for the evaluation of spondylolysis. Radiology 149: 315–316

McCulloch J A 1977 Chemonucleolysis. Journal of Bone and Joint Surgery 59–B: 45–52

McPhee I B, O'Brien J P 1979 Reduction of severe spondylolisthesis. Spine 4: 430–434

Maring-Klug R 1982 Reducing low back pain during pregnancy. Nurse Practitioner 7: 18–24

Murray Leslie C F, Lintott D J, Wright V 1977 The spone in sport and veteran military parachutists. Annals of Rheumatic Diseases 36: 332–342

Newman P H 1963 The etiology of spondylolisthesis. Journal of Bone and Joint Surgery, 45–B: 39–59

Porter R W, Park W 1982 Unilateral spondylolysis. Journal of Bone and Joint Surgery 64–B: 344–348

Roberts S, Beard H K, O'Brien J P 1982 Biochemical changes of intervertebral discs in patients with spondylolisthesis or with tears of the posterior annulus. Annals of the Rheumatic Diseases 41: 78–85

Roche M B, Rowe G G 1951 The incidence of separated neural arch and coincident bone variation: a survey of 4200 skeletons. Anat. Rec. 109: 233–252

Rowe G G, Roche M B 1953 The aetiology of separate neural arch. Journal of Bone and Joint Surgery 35–A: 102–110

Semon R L, Spengler D 1981 Significance of lumbar spondylolysis in college football players. Spine 6: 172–174

Stott J R R, Cyron B M, Hutton W C, Wall J C 1981 The mechanics of spondylolysis. Orthopaedic Mechanics Procedures and Devices, p 65–93, Academic Press, London, New York

Troup J D G 1975 Mechanical factors in spondylolisthesis and spondylolysis. Clinical Orthopaedics and Related Research 117: 59–67

Wiltse L L, Newman P H, Macnab I 1976 Classification of spondylolysis and spondylolisthesis. Clinical Orthopaedics and Related Research 117: 23–29

Wiltse L L, Jackson D W 1976 Treatment of spondylolisthesis and spondylolysis in children. Clinical Orthopaedics and Related Research 117: 92–100

Wiltse L, Glenn W, Spencer C, Porter I and Guyer R 1982 Alar transverse process impingement of the L.5 spinal nerve. (The Far Out Syndrome.) Presented to the International Society for the Study of the Lumbar Spine. Toronto.

Wiltse L L, Winter R B 1983 Terminology and measurement of spondylolisthesis. Journal of Bone and Joint Surgery 65–B: 768–772

17

Unilateral spondylolysis — patholgy, diagnosis and clinical significance

PATHOLOGY

Bilateral spondylolisthesis probably occurs in approximately five per cent of the population. In contrast, unilateral spondylolysis is rather rare. The classification of spondylolysis and spondylolisthesis by Wiltse, Newman and Macnab (1976) refers to bilateral lesions only and not to the unilateral defect. It has been reported by Stewart (1953) and was present in one-sixth of the spondylolytic specimens of Roche and Rowe (1951), one in four Willis' (1923), and one in three of Eisenstein's specimens (1978). We described the vertebral morphology of five specimens of unilateral spondylolysis (1982) each showing developmental asymmetry. The defect is more common on the right side (Willis, 1931). The pedicles and the superior apophyseal joints are in normal symmetrical relationship with the vertebral body (Fig. 17.1). There is, however, marked asymmetry of the neural arch, the inferior apophyseal joints and the posterior elements, (Fig. 17.2, 17.3). The

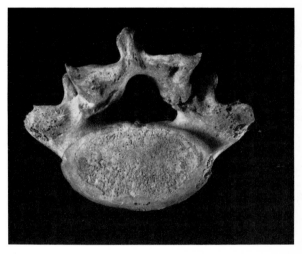

Fig. 17.2 Photograph of unilateral spondylolysis showing asymmetrically placed inferior apophyseal joints with the spinous process deviated away from the defective side.

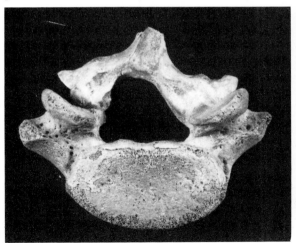

Fig. 17.1 Photograph of specimen with unilateral spondylolysis showing symmetrical superior apophyseal joints.

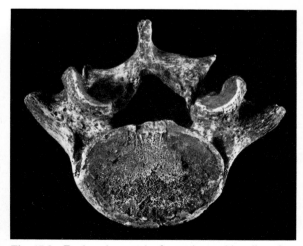

Fig. 17.3 Further photograph of a specimen with unilateral spondylolysis showing symmetrical superior apophyseal joints but asymmetrical inferior facets with deviation of the spinous process and asymmetrical vertebral canal.

combination of these effects produces a rotation of the spinous process away from the side of the lesion, the inferior apophyseal joint on that side being placed more dorsally than the superior. When viewed from behind, the neural arch is rotated in an anti-clockwise direction in the vertebra with a right sided defect, and clockwise in a left sided defect. The combined deformity results in horizontal orientation of the lamina on the affected side.

There is usually quite marked asymmetrical posterior wedging of the vertebral bodies, with reduction in the vertical height at the posterior angle of two to four millimetres.

Radiographs show that the areas of asymmetry are accompanied not only by a reduction in size of the lamina, apophyseal joint and transverse process, but also by thinner cortices and fewer trabeculae in these locations (Fig. 17.4). Posterior asymmetrical wedging of the vertebral body is shown in Fig. 17.5 and this is accompanied by a tendency to horizontal orientation of the pars interarticularis and the inferior apophyseal joint on the affected side. The spondylolytic defects vary in width which determines the facility with which they can be demonstrated radiologically. A defect of one millimetre cannot be demonstrated by an axial projection, even when using thin section computerised tomography.

DIAGNOSIS

Although unilateral spondylolysis may well occur in a little less than one per cent of the population, its

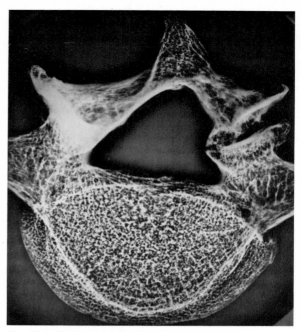

Fig. 17.4   Radiograph of unilateral spondylolysis.

detection is extremely difficult. We seldom make the diagnosis of unilateral spondylolyis in clinical practice. This may be because it rarely produces symptoms. The wide dome-shaped vertebral canal produced by elongation of the pars, albeit asymmetrical widening, does protect the neural elements from compression in the presence of disc pathology, degenerative change, and segmental

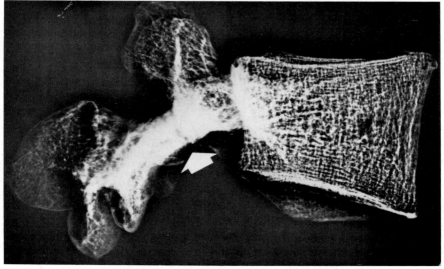

Fig. 17.5   Radiograph of the same specimen showing marked asymmetrical wedging of the vertebral body.

movement. In addition, the intact, thickened unilateral pars does resist shear, and avoids the instability that can accompany bilateral defects. Alternatively, we may fail to recognise unilateral defects because we do not suspect them, and even if suspected, they are extremely difficult to demonstrate radiologically. It may be suspected when there is asymmetrical postero-lateral wedging of the vertebral body, horizontal orientation of the lamina or hypoplasia of one inferior apophyseal facet. However, even computerised tomography may not always reveal the defect. Radiographs taken at a 45 degree oblique angle, with the tube inclined 20 degrees cranially may be of help (Fig. 17.6) and may give some additional information about hypertrophic bone indenting the root canal. Because of these difficulties in visualisation, it is possible that unilateral spondylolysis is more frequent than is generally acknowledged.

AETIOLOGICAL SIGNIFICANCE

It is difficult to reconcile the morphological finding of unilateral spondylolysis with the various theories on the aetiology of bilateral spondylolysis. Opinions vary on the cause of the lytic defect in the pars interarticularis. The major controversy centres on the dilemma of whether the defects are congenital or traumatic. A number of authors (Newman, 1963, Farfan, 1973, and Troup 1975, 1977) have felt that the two are not mutually incompatible, and that an individual may be congenitally predisposed to a stress

fracture of the pars. Undoubtedly, fractures of the pars may be seen to heal (Devas, 1963, Murray and Colwill, 1968, Krenz and Troup 1973, Jackson, Wiltse and Cirincone, 1976). Specimens of unilateral spondylolysis, however, do not show any evidence of a healed fracture on the side opposite the defect, nor of attempted healing of the unilateral lysis. It would be unlikely for a single fracture to occur in a ring of bone like the neural arch, and if a double fracture occurred, it would be unusual for one of the fractures alone to heal. The very existence of unilateral spondylolysis must question the concept that spondylolysis is always the result of a stress fracture.

The morphological changes in unilateral spondlolysis with unilateral asymmetry and hypoplasia, provide some understanding of the changes that are observed in bilateral spondylolysis. At least some features are common in both unilateral and bilateral conditions. Wedging of the vertebral body occurs with bilateral lysis, and unilateral wedging of the body with unilateral lysis. Both laminae are orientated horizontally with the bilateral defect, and one lamina asymmetrically orientated in the horizontal plane with the unilateral defect. In an isolated specimen of unilateral spondylolysis, the most obvious deformity is asymmetry of the neural arch, with deviation of the spinous process away from the side having the hypoplastic elements. In the articulated spine, however, the spinous processes may maintain a mid-line position. This could only occur with forward rotation of the vertebra on the affected side, and result in a hemilisthesis. It is probable that the asymmetrical morphological changes occur before

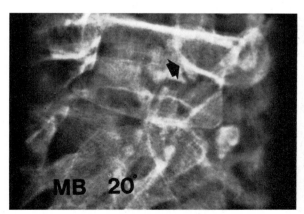

Fig. 17.6A An oblique radiograph with a 20 degree incline showing the unilateral defect on the left side.

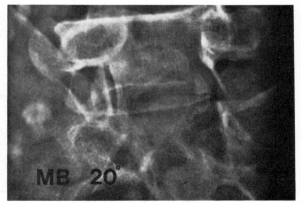

Fig. 17.6B A 20 degree inclined plane on the unaffected side shows no abnormality.

skeletal maturity is complete, and that the changes are a growth phenomenon. If we extrapolate to the bilateral situation, all the characteristics of bilateral spondylolisthesis are present, with elongation of the pars, horizontal orientation of the laminae, and olisthesis and wedging of the vertebral body. Thus the changes recorded in unilateral spondylolysis suggest that many of the changes in bilateral spondylolisthesis are a growth phenomenon.

There is histological evidence that growth remodelling occurs in the posterior elements. Park et al (1980) have studied the changes in grossly displaced adolescent spondylolisthesis. This revealed pronounced elongation of the pars interarticularis as a result of remodelling secondarily to the stress loading. It was accompanied by underdevelopment of the posterior elements, notably of the inferior facets.

CLINICAL SIGNIFICANCE

The clinical implications of unilateral spondylolysis

must remain speculative. Possible factors could include the effects of unilateral rotation, with torsional damage to the intervertebral disc, and disturbance of the nerve root (Farfan et al, 1970), which could then be aggravated by hypertrophic bone projecting into the nerve root canal. A significant contributory factor is likely to be the presence of spina bifida which will produce a free floating fragment, and thereby contribute to segmental instability.

As with bilateral spondylolisthesis, the absence of the trefoil configuration ensures that even with a compromising lesion, the neural contents in the central canal are protected. The fifth lumbar root is probably more vulnerable, however, in the root canal. It is only as we become more proficient in diagnosing unilateral spondylolysis, that the full clinical implications will be revealed. However, it should be specifically sought in patients with asymmetrical vertebral wedging and associated hypoplasia of the neural arch.

REFERENCES

Devas M B 1963 Stress fractures in children. Journal of Bone and Joint Surgery 45–B: 528–541
Eisenstein S M C 1978 Spondylolysis. A skeletal investigation of two population groups. Journal of Bone and Joint Surgery: 60–B: 488–494
Farfan H F, Cossette J W, Robertson G H, Wells R V, Kraus H 1970 The effects of torsion on the lumbar intervertebral joints: the role of torsion in the production of disc degeneration. Journal of Bone and Joint Surgery 52–A: 468–497
Farfan H F 1973 The mechanical disorders of the lower back. Philadelphia, Lea and Febiger
Jackson D W, Wiltse L L, Cirincone R J 1976 Spondylolysis in the female gymnast. Clinical Orthopaedics 117: 68–73
Krenz J, Troup J D G 1973 The structure of the pars interarticularis of the lower lumbar vertebrae and its relation to the aetiology of spondylolysis with a report of the healing fracture in the neural arch of a fourth lumbar vertebrae. Journal of Bone and Joint Surgery 55–B: 735–741
Murray R O, Colwill M R 1968 Stress fractures of the pars interarticularis. Proceedings of the Royal Society of Medicine 61: 555–557
Newman P H 1963 The etiology of spondylolisthesis. Journal of Bone and Joint Surgery 45–B: 39–59

Park W M, Webb J K, O'Brien J P, McCall I W 1980 The microstructure of the neural arch complex in adolescence: a histological and radiological correlation in spondylolisthesis. Proceeding of the Institute of Mechanical Engineering 35–36
Porter R W, Park W, 1982 Unilateral spondylolysis. Journal of Bone and Joint Surgery 45–B: 39–59
Roche M B, Rowe G G 1951 The incidence of separated neural arch and coincident bone variations: a survey of 4200 skeletons. Anat Rec. 109: 233–252
Stewart T D 1953 The age-incidence of neural arch defects in Alaskan natives, considering the standpoint of aetiology. Journal of Bone and Joint Surgery 35–A: 937–950
Troup J D G 1975 Mechanical factors in spondylolisthesis and spondylolysis. Clinical Orthopaedics and Related Research 117: 59–67
Troup J D G 1977 The etiology of spondylolsis. Orthopaedic Clinics of North America 81: 57–64
Willis T A 1923 The lumbo-sacral vertebral column in man, its stability of form and function. American Journal of Anatomy 32: 95–123
Willis T A 1931 The seperate neural arch. Journal of Bone and Joint Surgery 13: 709–721
Wiltse L L, Newman P H, Macnab I 1976 Classification of spondylolysis and spondylolisthesis. Clinical Orthopaedics and Related Research 117: 23–29

18

Degenerative spondylolisthesis — pathology, symptoms and management

PATHOLOGY

Forward displacement of a proximal vertebra in relation to its adjacent vertebra when associated with an intact neural arch, no congenital anomaly and in the presence of degenerative change, is known as 'degenerative spondylolisthesis' (Wiltse, Newman and Macnab, 1976). It was described by Junghanns (1931) and Schmorl and Junghanns (1932) who noted that it was more common in women, and often occurred between the fourth and fifth lumbar vertebrae. This contrasts with isthmic spondylolisthesis (Table 18.1).

The displacement, when it occurs, begins in the sixth decade, and patients generally attend with symptoms around sixty years of age (Newman, 1963). The displacement is limited, and a slip ratio of more than 15 per cent is unusual (Junghanns, 1930, Macnab, 1950).

Forward displacement results from a failure of the apophyseal joints to restrain shear. They are orientated in the sagittal plane in the upper lumbar spine, and become progressively more coronally orientated towards the lower lumbar spine (Table 6.1, page 40).

The increasing shear forces in the lower lumbar lordotic spine are balanced by the progressively efficient restraint of the coronally orientated lower lumbar facets. L.4/5 appears to be the level where the joints may fail to restrain shear.

There are several possible factors causing this failure:

1. Constitutional variation in the orientation of the apophyseal joints. Those individuals whose L.4/5 facets are more sagittaly orientated than the rest of the population will be more prone to displacement.

2. The mechanical strength of the subchondral bone. The osteoporotic spine will be vulnerable to microfractures, with deformity of the facets. It had been suggested that an increased angle between the pedicle and inferior articular facet would allow forward subluxation of the upper vertebra (Junghann, 1930 and Macnab, 1950), but Newman (1963) found no increase of this angle in the slipping vertebra. He did suspect that progressive widening of the angle may accompany the progressive slip from remodelling in response to microscopic stress fractures.

3. A degenerate disc will less effectively restrain shear (Larson, 1983).

4. An increased lumbar lordosis will increase the force of shear but there is no evidence that these patients have an increased lumbo sacral angle (Table 18.2). Posture, especially in pregnancy when the

Table 18.1 Comparison between the segmental level and sex ratio in degenerative and isthmic spondylolisthesis.

	Degenerative Spondylolisthesis (n−53)	Isthmic Spondylolisthesis (n−107)
Percentage Male	22%	57%
L.3/4	12%	2%
L.4/5	78%	15%
L.5/S.1	12%	85%

Table 18.2 Mean lumbo sacral angle for patients with degenerative spondylolisthesis, isthmic spondylolisthesis and other patients with back pain.

	Mean lumbo-sacral angle.
Degenerative spondylolisthesis (n−58)	30.8° (±7.1°)
Isthmic spondylolisthesis (n−107)	37.3° (±8.3°)
Other patients with low back pain (n−60)	30.3° (±6.4°)

ligamentous restraint is less effective, is probably significant.

5. Poor spinal and abdominal muscles place proportionally greater strain on the apophyseal joints. Newman believed that the facets give way from an acquired instability of the soft tissues (1963) especially the interspinous and supraspinous ligaments, and he thought the high incidence of spina bifida occulta important. There is no evidence that these patients have generalised ligamentous-joint laxity.

6. Obesity, disproportionate to muscle strength, increases the shear.

Several of these factors in combination may explain the higher incidence of degenerative spondylolisthesis in women.

The proximal vertebra steadily displaces forwards, deforming the vertebral canal, the root canal and the intervertebral formainae (Fig. 18.1). If the central canal is already constitutionally narrow, then vertebral displacement with an intact neural arch will

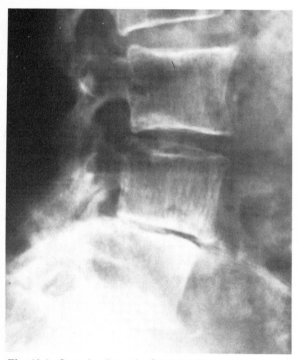

Fig. 18.1 Lateral radiograph of patient with degenerative spondylolisthesis at L.4/5. The disc space is reduced with bony sclerosis and forward displacement of the body of L.4, with an intact neural arch. There is deformity of the superior facet of L.5 and deformation of the central canal, root canal and intervertebral foramen.

deform the dura and its contents. The root canal can also become critically narrow, especially at the foraminal exit. If a dynamic element is superimposed on the reduction of space for the neural contents, pathological changes develop in the dura and nerve roots, producing symptoms.

The proximal vertebra may be displaced and yet in a neutral equilibrium; that is, movement may not cause further displacement beyond the limits of normal restraint. Alternatively, it may be displaced and unstable, being further displaced by movement beyond the normal limits of restraint. This is a theoretical distinction, but it does have practical implications. A vertebra which has displaced but has reached a position of neutral equilibrium, is unlikely to produce symptons of fatigue in the soft tissues which restrain shear, nor momentary subluxation pain in the apophyseal joints or dura. A displaced vertebra with a degree of associated unnatural segmental movement may produce either of these symptoms.

Degenerative changes develop in the apophyseal joints and at the margins of the vertebral bodies, until a degree of stability occurs. These osteophytic changes can encroach into the root canal. It is interesting that the vertebral body does not become wedge-shaped as in the displaced body of an isthmic spondylolisthesis, the former displacing in adult life, the latter during growth.

SYMPTOMS ASSOCIATED WITH DEGENERATIVE SPONDYLOLISTHESIS.

The anatomical displacement of one vertebra upon another does not necessarily cause symptoms. If they do occur, it is generally the result of embarrassment of the dura and nerve roots within a small deformed central canal or root canal.

Symptoms of instability

1. Momentary subluxation pain is a common symptom, with discomfort rising from the stooped position or getting up out of a chair. Patients will support the trunk with the hands on their thighs as they stand up after stooping. Sudden movements, and turning in bed can be painful. Standing and walking causes fatigue pain, with aching in the back and thighs. It is relieved by rest. Flexion is not limited,

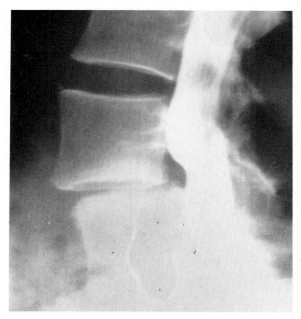

Fig. 18.2A A radiculogram of a patient with degenerative spondylolisthesis at L.4/5 with distortion of the metrizamide column in extension.

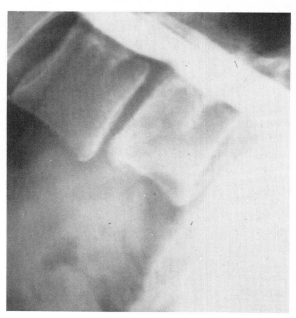

Fig. 18.2B The anterior dural deformation is largely corrected in flexion.

and they can frequently place the flat of the hands on the floor. They may have an extension catch and no lumbar extension. Tenderness is localised to the level of the displacement. There are no abnormal neurological signs unless there is another associated lesion.

The mechanism of these instability symptoms is speculative. Some believe that the apophyseal joints are probably the pain source, but this does not explain why some patients with degenerative spondylolisthesis are quite symptom free. Our ultrasound measurement of the vertebral canal in 81 patients with back pain and degenerative spondylolisthesis suggest that some have narrow central canals, the mean measurement at L.5 being 1.39 cm (SD .08 cm.). If the canal size is a relevant factor, then the momentary subluxating pain may be dural in origin (Fig. 18.2).

2. The L.4 root within its root canal is at risk in an L.4/5 degenerative spondylolisthesis. It can produce the classical symptoms of root entrapment (page 106) but the pain may be particularly influenced by posture and by spinal rotation. The L.5 root is vulnerable as it crosses a rolled rim of L.4/5 disc (Fig. 18.3).

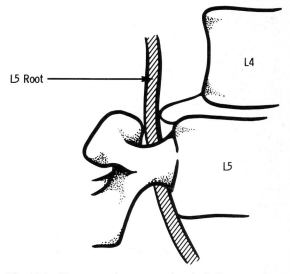

Fig. 18.3 Diagram to demonstrate that the L.5 root can be affected in the central canal from a rim of L.4/5 disc in degenerative spondylolisthesis.

3. Neurogenic claudication can be precipitated by a degenerative spondylolisthesis, especially in men. It is not common in women, but about half the male patients with neurogenic claudication have some

vertebral displacement with an intact neural arch. A pre-existing narrow canal with some forward vertebral displacement is an unpleasant combination.

MANAGEMENT OF SYMPTOMS ASSOCIATED WITH DEGENERATIVE SPONDYLOLISTHESIS

Instability pain is effectively managed with an explanation of the pain mechanism, and appropriate advice. Pain in the back, perhaps referred to the buttocks and thighs, is seldom so severe that a conservative approach is not adequate. They are helped by the 'back school' programme, when fitness and obesity are discussed. Lifting is demonstrated and practised, avoiding stooping and twisting. They are reassured that with time and the inevitable stiffness of the years, their unstable spinal segment should become more stable and less troublesome.

Root entrapment syndrome can usually be managed conservatively, though occasionally the severity, disability and duration of the pain makes surgical intervention necessary. It may not be possible to recognise pre-operatively which nerve root is involved. The clinical examination may help with support from E.M.G. studies and a CT scan but it may only be at the time of operation that the correct root is identified after adequate decompression and exposure.

Removal of the lamina usually reveals an hour-glass constriction of the dura, compressed from either side by osteophytic outgrowths of the apophyseal joint. The L.4 root can be involved in the deformed root canal, and it needs complete decompression well laterally removing much of the inferior and superior facets of the apophyseal joints on the affected side. Provided the joint is not completely removed, and that the contralateral joint is undisturbed, there is no real risk of subsequent increase in the vertebral displacement (Epstein et al 1983).

The L.5 root can be involved in the central canal as it passes over the ridged L.4/5 disc. There is counter compression dorsally from the cranial edge of the lamina of L.5. Attempts to remove the thickened rim of L.4/5 disc are not usually very successful, and removal of the posterior vertebral bar of L.5 is likewise difficult. Decompression of the central canal by removal of the L.5 lamina does, however, provide more space for the L.5 root. The L.5 root is often kinked in the lateral recess of a trefoil shaped central canal, under and overlapping superior facet. The medial edge of the facet must be excised and the facet undercut to effectively decompress the root.

The treatment of neurogenic claudication is discussed in chapter 14 but if surgical decompression is attempted in the presence of degenerative spondylolisthesis, it is important to leave a remnant of the inferior facets to prevent further subluxation of the displaced vertebra. It is more likely that we shall fail to relieve symptoms because of an inadequate decompression, than produce symptoms from further displacement.

REFERENCES

Epstein N E, Epstein J A, Carras R and Lavine L S 1983 Degenerative spondylolisthesis with an intact neural arch; a review of 60 cases with analysis of clinical findings and the development of surgical management. Neurosurgery 13: 555–561

Junghanns H 1930 Spondylolisthesen ohne Spalt im zwischengelenkstuck. Archiv fur Orthopadische und Unfall Chirurgie 29: 118

Larson S J 1983 Degenerative spondylolisthesis. Neurosurgery 13: 561

Macnab I 1950 Spondylolisthesis with an intact neural arch so called pseudospondylolisthesis. Journal of Bone and Joint Surgery 32–B: 325

Newman P H 1963 The etiology of spondylolisthesis. Journal of Bone and Joint Surgery 45–B: 39–59

Schmorl G, Junghanns H 1932 Die gesunde und krande wirbelsaule. Leipzig. George Thieme

Wiltse L L, Newman P H, Macnab I 1976 Classification of spondylolysis and spondylolisthesis. Clinical Orthopaedics and Related Research 117: 23–29

19

Retrolisthesis and rotational displacement — patholgy and clinical significance

PATHOLOGY

Vertebral displacement can occur in any one of the three axes of rotation, sagittal, coronal or transverse, (Fig. 19.1). Retrolisthesis implies a posterior displacement of the proximal vertebral body in the sagittal plane, but in practise, it is more often in two or even three planes (Farfan, 1973). A single radiograph in the lateral projection may show what appears to be a posterior displacement (Fig. 19.2) and this may indeed be confirmed in the absence of lateral and rotational displacement in the antero-posterior view.

The lateral radiograph, however, often gives a hint of a combined rotational displacement, by the double shadow of the posterior vertebral body margin (Fig. 19.3). The asymmetrical facets in the antero-posterior film suggests a rotational element in the displacement. If the facets are symmetrical the vertebra will displace posteriorly but asymmetrical facets will cause rotational displacement (Cyron and Hutton, 1980). Unequal facet degeneration may produce asymmetry, with remodelling from stress and microfracture, and subsequent rotational

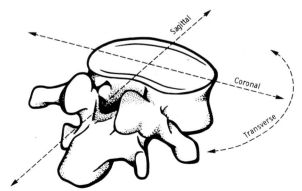

Fig. 19.1 Diagram to show axes of rotation.

displacement. Malalignment of the spinous processes also supports a rotational element to the vertebral displacement (Fig. 19.4).

Retrolisthesis, with posterior and/or rotational displacement is the result of disc degeneration, loss of disc height, and the shingling effect of the apophyseal joints (Chandnani and Chhabria, 1978). It usually occurs at L.4/5 or L.3/4 level (Fig. 19.5).

Whether the displacement is posterior, rotational or lateral, the vertebral canal and its contents may be compromised. The dura is vulnerable in a small central canal, with change in spinal posture causing dural irritation, (Fig. 19.6). Neurogenic claudication is unusual.

The nerve root is at risk in the root canal and at the foramen. The effects of the displacement is compounded by bony and soft tissue degenerative change around the apophyseal joints, and by the formation of a posterior vertebral bar and ridging of the disc annulus. Then a rotatory movement or lateral flexion at the level of displacement, further reduces the cross sectional area of the foramen.

When space is critically limited, it is the combination of change of posture, and nerve root excursion, that produces pathological changes in the root, with symptoms of root entrapment.

Retrolisthesis rarely causes symptoms in the upper lumbar spine where the canal and foramina are more spacious. It is lower lumbar displacement, with associated pathological changes, that affects the neural elements.

CLINICALLY

The majority of patients attending with retrolisthesis are middle aged men with a decade of previous back pain. There are two common syndromes.

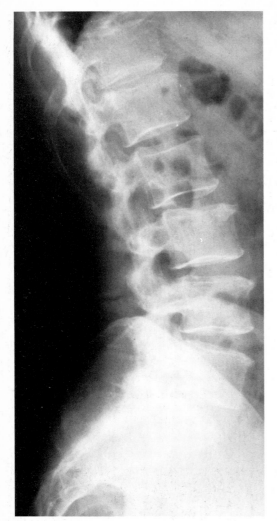

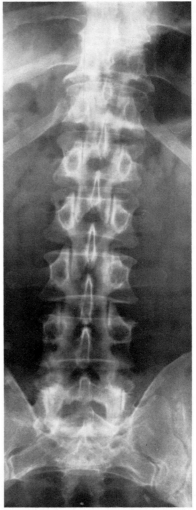

Fig. 19.2A Lateral radiograph showing posterior displacement of L.2 on L.3, and L.3 on L.4 with traction spurs.

Fig. 19.2B An antero-posterior radiograph confirms that the displacement is mainly in the sagittal plane. The apophyseal joints are symmetrical, sagittally orientated, and the spinous processes in the mid line with no rotation.

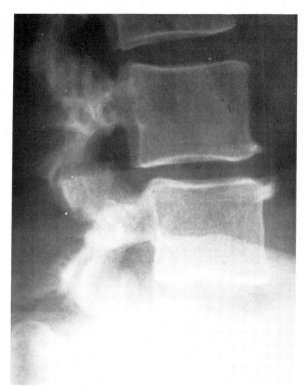

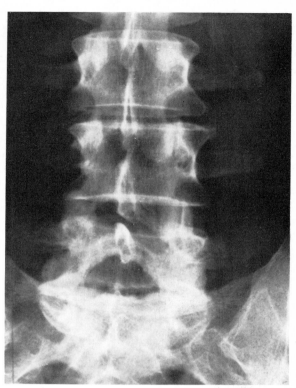

Fig. 19.3A Lateral radiograph showing disc space narrowing, traction spurs and posterior displacement of the body of L.3. A double shadow of the posterior border of L.3 suggests a combined rotational displacement in the transverse plane.

Fig. 19.3B An antero-posterior radiograph of the same patient shows asymmetrical apophyseal joints at L.3/4 and some displacement of the body of L.3 in the coronal plane.

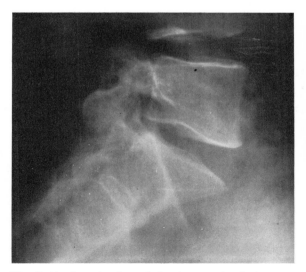

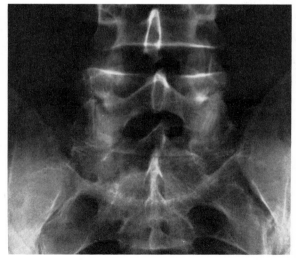

Fig. 19.4A Lateral radiograph showing posterior displacement of the body of L.4.

Fig. 19.4B An antero posterior radiograph of the same patient shows asymmetrical apophyseal joints at L.4/5 and malalignment of the spinous process of L.4.

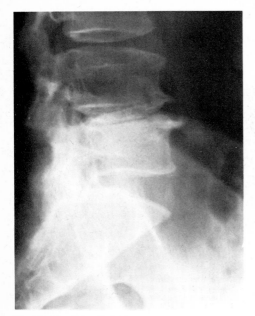

Fig. 19.5A   Retrolisthesis at L.4/5 level.

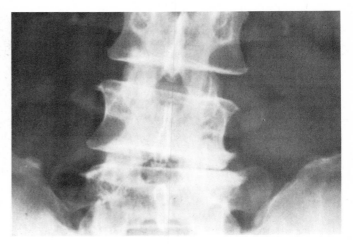

Fig. 19.5B   Antero posterior view shows that this is also partially a rotational displacement.

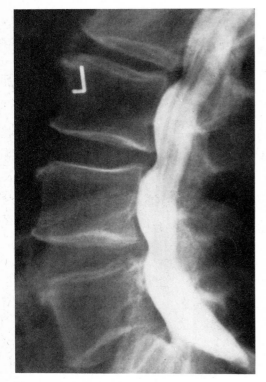

Fig. 19.6A   Lateral radiculogram of extended spine in a patient with some retrolisthesis at L.3/4 level.

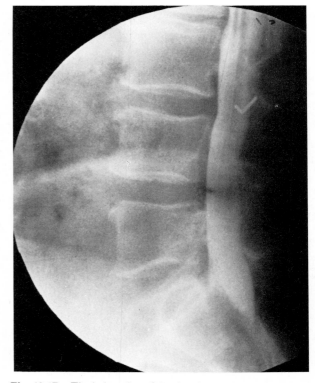

Fig. 19.6B   The indentation of the dura is corrected in flexion.

1. Root entrapment

Forty-two per cent of our 177 patients attending with a retro (or rotational) listhesis, had root pain below the knee incriminating a single nerve. Displacement at L.4 can affect the fourth root in the root canal, or the fifth root in the central canal, over a posterior vertebral bar, or beneath a superior facet. L.3 displacement can similarly affect the third or fourth root. The root pain is affected by spinal posture, or rarely root claudication pain relieved by rest. It is not the major cause of root entrapment, but when displacement does occur, the root is at risk (Fig. 13.4).

2. Posture related back pain

It is an important factor in posture related back pain in the middle aged and elderly, either from dural irritation or apophyseal joint pain.

In both of these syndromes, limited spinal flexion is not a feature of the examination, but probably because extension further limits the space in the central and root canal, this is reduced or absent. Space seems to be highly significant in the causation of symptoms. Nearly half of our 177 patients with retrolisthesis had ultrasound measurement of the central canal below the tenth percentile for asymptomatic subjects.

Spinal tenderness is localised to the site of the lesion, and firm rotatory pressure on the spinous process may reproduce the root pain (door-bell sign).

TREATMENT

The patient has learnt that symptoms are related to certain movements and to posture. A change of posture when pain develops, and avoidance of movements that cause pain, is obvious advice to be reinforced in a back school by an explanation of ways of reducing spinal stress in everyday life. A corset with a frame rather than parallel steels, can help by restricting rotation and lateral flexion. It should be accompanied by advice about maintaining good muscle strength from swimming and walking. Severe root pain may require epidural injections.

A few patients need surgical help, involving unilateral root canal decompression for root entrapment, and bilateral decompression for back pain. Every effort should be made to identify the affected root before surgery. The lesion may be too distal for identification by myelography, and although CT scan may show bony encroachment, this is not necessarily the site of the lesion. The root may be recognised at operation from its size, its colour, its consistency and perhaps more significantly from its tension.

If the root is affected in the central canal, bilateral decompression is advisable, removing part of the rolled ridged annulus at the level of displacement. Involvement in the root canal requires adequate decompression with undercutting of the superior facet on the affected side and a major part of the apophyseal joint.

REFERENCES

Chandnani P G, Chhabria P B 1978 Posterior spinal compression by the cephalad edge of the laminae and its role in the etiology of backache. Neurology India 26: 7–9

Cyron B M, Hutton W C 1980 Articular trophism and stability of the lumbar spine. Spine 5: 168–172
Farfan H F 1973 The mechanical disorders of the lower back. Philadelphia, Lea and Febiger

20

Compression fractures of the vertebral bodies — pathology, symptoms, natural history, management

PATHOLOGY

Compression fractures of the thoracic and lumbar vertebral bodies are usually the result of a vertical compression force. They may result from a fall from a height, a weight falling on the shoulders, or conversely from a vertical force such as a pilot's ejector seat or an exploding mine at sea.

T.12, L.1 and L.2 are the vertebral bodies most frequently fractured, with a decreasing incidence proximally and distally (Nicoll, 1949, Young, 1973). Two or more vertebrae may be fractured, not necessarily adjacent to each other. The deformity of the vertebral body resulting from the compression is variable and sometimes asymmetrical. CT scans show how much more extensive is the fracture than suggested from conventional radiographs; the posterior cortex is not always intact. The anterior cortex fails, and sometimes also the superior vertebral end plate. The degree of deformity in the sagittal plane can be measured from the angle of the upper and lower borders of the vertebral body on a lateral radiograph, or as a ratio of the anterior over the posterior vertebral body depth (Young, 1973).

Provided that the posterior elements avoid injury, it is unusual to have neurological damage (Holdsworth, 1963). This is not absolute, because if the vertebral canal is already narrow, a flexion deformity that accompanies a compression fracture may cause critical compression of the spinal cord and paraplegia. Occasionally neurological symptoms develop in later years (Fig. 20.1). Generally, however, compression of the vertebral body without bony injury to the pedicles, facets or isthmus is not considered a serious injury. There is no neurological injury, and the stability of the spine is not affected.

Some patients, in addition to the vertebral body

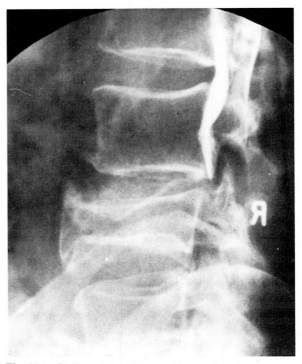

Fig. 20.1 Radiograph of a 73 year old man with a 5 year history of neurogenic claudication and 16 years of back pain following compression fracture of the body of L.4. There was a pre-existing shallow vertebral canal. The metrizamide does not flow below L.3/4.

fracture, also damage one of the intervertebral discs. This is frequently missed clinically, being overshadowed by the more obvious bony injury, but persisting symptoms in the lower lumbar region make this associated injury suspect. Adams and Hutton (1982) have shown that experimental disc compression in flexion can injure the annulus and cause disc prolapse. This may be more significant in an injury to a previously damaged annulus.

Our studies of 71 patients who had sustained compression fractures of the spine, recorded a correlation between the persistence of symptoms and the size of the vertebral canal (Table 20.1). Whether the persisting pain source was at the site of fracture or from a more distal disc lesion is uncertain.

Table 20.1 Relationship between ultrasound measurement of the vertebral canal and persistence of back pain symptoms in 71 patients following vertebral compression fracture (mean time after fracture 4.4 years)
Significant difference between groups 1 and 2 at L.5 ($p < 0.02$)

	28 patients with no symptoms or very mild occasional back pain not limiting activities.	26 patients with intermittent back pain affecting activities.	17 patients with severe or constant back and or leg pain.
L.1	1.50	1.48	1.47
L.2	1.46	1.45	1.44
L.3	1.45	1.42	1.41
L.4	1.42	1.40	1.39
L.5	1.43	1.39	1.38

SYMPTOMS

Symptoms at the time of the fracture are variable in degree and are not related to the severity of compression (Nicholl, 1949, Young, 1973). A few patients are able to keep on their feet, but most have severe pain in the back at the site of injury. Retroperitoneal or mediastinal bleeding adds to the discomfort. Abnormal neurological signs are rare, if the fracture involves the vertebral body only. The tenderness is well localised to the level of fracture, an important sign if a patient presents with acute back pain and the tenderness is not at the level of the wedged vertebra. Such a compressed vertebra is a fossil of some long forgotten injury.

MANAGEMENT

Bed rest is advisable until a reduction in pain allows mobilisation in reasonable comfort. This may take a few days, or a couple of weeks. Graded mobility is encouraged. There is no evidence that either long periods of bed rest, or early energetic exercises influence the recovery. What is probably more important is a careful explanation of the significance of the fractured vertebra. It is reassuring for the patient to know that they should eventually become symptom free, and when pain does persist, it is usually intermittent and not disabling. A corset is usually unnecessary. Plenty of walking and swimming is encouraged in the recovery period.

NATURAL HISTORY

If patients with a litigation problem are excluded, then the majority with vertebral compression fractures become free of symptoms within a few months of injury. Litigation influences the natural history considerably. This may be because these injuries result from industrial and road accidents, generally with more violence than domestic accidents. Alternatively, the financial implications associated with litigation may generate genuine distress and abnormal pain behaviour.

Our studies of 71 patients up to 10 years after the fracture, suggest that when back pain does persist it becomes less troublesome with time. This corresponds with the observation that relatively few patients with a previous compression fracture seek help with back pain later in life.

COMPRESSION FRACTURE OF THE SPINE FROM SKELETAL FAILURE

Although there is no precise information about the incidence of vertebral compression fractures due to skeletal failure, extrapolation from clinical surveys suggests that about 2.5 per cent of women are affected by 60 years of age, and 7.5 per cent by 80 years of age (Nordin et al, 1980). Such fractures are much less common in men.

The commonest cause of spinal skeletal failure is osteoporosis, where there is a deficiency in bone mass per unit volume. The bone present is essentially normal, but the mass reduced.

Age, sex and especially the menopause, are important in the development of osteoporosis, but bone mass may be reduced by immobilisation, corticosteroid drugs, hyperparathyroidism, Cushing's syndrome, hypogonadism, and by bone replacement by myelomatosis, reticuloendothelial disorders and these need to be excluded before one can assume that a compression fracture in the elderly is the result of the more common age-related (senile) osteoporosis.

Osteomalacia, where the bone mass is reduced, with decreased mineralisation of the osteoid, may coexist with osteoporosis and also needs to be excluded. It is probably frequently unrecognised. In engineering terms, failure due to poor design is more common than failure from inefficient material. Probably also in skeletal failure, abnormal bony architecture related to osteomalacia is as common as insufficient bone mass alone.

The degree of osteoporosis is probably related to bone stock developed in earlier life, and the rate of bone loss thereafter. The rate of cortical bone loss is comparable in males and females (0.5–1 per cent per annum) but because men have a greater initial bone mass, the amount of bone remaining in men is greater than in women. Trabecular bone loss is probably related to lack of ovarian function, and thus after the menopause, the superimposition of increased trabecular loss increases the risk of skeletal failure in the trabecular bones of women. In crush fractures of the vertebral bodies, there is unequivocal deficiency of trabecular bone if assessed by iliac crest bone biopsy (Nordin, 1983).

We know little about the matrix and this in addition to osteoporosis may hold the key to skeletal failure.

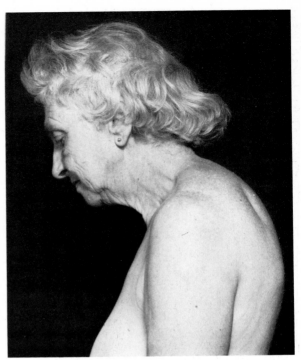

Fig. 20.2   Kyphotic posture of a woman with vertebral osteoporosis.

Clinically

One or several vertebral bodies may collapse suddenly or slowly. Sudden failure of one vertebral body results in spontaneous severe back pain. It becomes easier, settling over several weeks, unless another vertebra collapses. Gradual failure of several vertebrae is often associated with chronic back pain, sometimes with episodic increase in the pain with development of a kyphosis, the 'dowager's hump' and loss of height (Fig. 20.2). Abdominal skin folds appear, and with gross collapse, the ribs can rest on the iliac crest.

After a recent fracture, there is localised tenderness to pressure over the spinous process, and muscle spasm.

A patient may present with cervical symptoms from a compensatory cervical lordosis, rather than with a painful thoracic spine, or alternatively with low back pain. The centre of gravity is thrown forwards by the upper thoracic kyphosis and in attempting to compensate for this, the lumbar spine extends. This can disturb the apophyseal joints, cause impingement of the spinous process, and if space in the vertebral

canal is at a premium, the neural elements can be embarrassed. There is some evidence that in contrast to men whose peak incidence of back pain is at 40 years of age, there is a steadily increasing incidence of back pain in women with advancing age (Fin Biering-Sorensen, 1982) and it is tempting to speculate that menopausal osteoporosis is partly responsible.

Investigations

The clinical diagnosis is confirmed radiologically. One or more vertebrae are collapsed, with loss of mineral content appearing as decreased density. The trabecular bone may become almost radiolucent, and the cortical shell give the appearance of a 'ghost vertebra'. In the thoracic spine, collapse of the vertebral body is mainly at the anterior aspect, producing the kyphus. The intervertebral discs develop a biconcave appearance as subcortical microfractures permit the disc to encroach into the adjacent vertebrae, described as 'cod fish vertebrae' (Resnick, 1982) (Fig. 20.3). The radiological signs are not always so apparent, because one-third of the

The patient whose initial severe pain is now settling down, is more likely to have age-related skeletal failure, than the patient whose back pain is steadily getting worse. The latter needs thorough investigation.

Biochemical assays have proved of little value in the diagnosis of osteoporosis, apart from excluding other conditions. In osteomalacia blood test may show low to normal calcium and phosphorus and raised alkaline phosphatase but a bone biopsy is necessary for confirmation. Facilities for photon-absorption densiometry to measure bone density and neutron activation analysis to measure total body calcium, are available in but few centres. Ultrasound has the potential to measure bone density and possibly bony architecture (Langton et al, 1984) (Fig. 20.4) and may prove to be useful in quantitating osteoporosis.

Management

The sudden severe pain of a collapsed vertebra does require a few days rest in bed, but because of increased bone loss associated with recumbency, this should be for a minimum of time. Early mobilisation

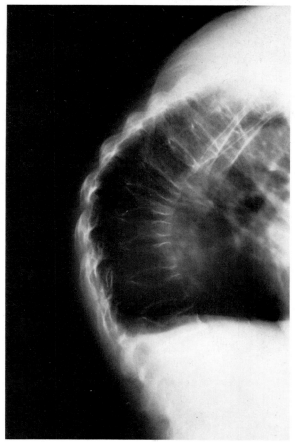

Fig. 20.3 Lateral radiograph of an osteoporotic thoracic spine with several compression fractures and biconcave appearance of the intervertebral discs.

skeletal mass is lost before there is bone rarifaction on the plain radiograph (Stevenson and Whitehead, 1982).

Most patients with skeletal failure of the vertebral bodies have age-related ostoporosis, and because active treatment is of doubtful value, too much investigation for an elderly patient is not justified. Investigations are necessary, however, if there is a suspicion that the demineralisation can be treated, or if there are signs of osteomalacia.

Is there a past history of gastric surgery, with the possibility of deficient dietary intake and poor absorption? Is there evidence of renal disease or biliary cirrhosis? Is she receiving corticosteroids? Is there evidence of hyperparathyroidism? Is there a blood dyscrasia, or a suggestion of skeletal metastases? Are there radiological loozer zones?

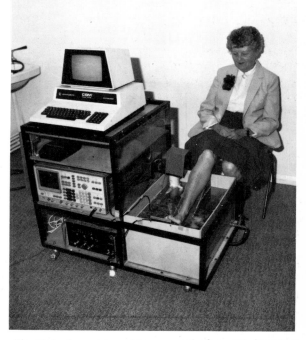

Fig. 20.4 Apparatus used to measure the frequency dependant attenuation of ultrasound across the os calcis.

and activity is encouraged. In fact, exercise is the only known way of reducing the rate of demineralisation. A word of encouragement that the pain will slowly settle is appreciated. Corsets are unhelpful and tend to be more cumbersome than useful.

The slowly developing kyphus of several collapsing vertebrae cannot be prevented by a support though a brace is often requested. Mobilisation techniques should be avoided, lest they precipitate further injury.

Impingement of the twelfth rib on the iliac crest can be a troublesome source of back pain, when it is difficult to palpate between the rib and the pelvis in the seated patient. The offending rib is tender and its excision can produce welcome relief (Fig. 20.5).

At present there is no sure way of reducing the rate of demineralisation in osteoporosis, let alone replace bone. It is worth ensuring that there is an adequate dietary intake of calcium and vitamin D but supplements are unnecessary if the diet is adequate. There is no good evidence that oral calcium supplement can prevent post-menopausal and senile osteoporosis (Stevenson and Whitehead, 1983). Several therapeutic regimes have been shown to reduce demineralisation, some even to increase total body calcium, including hormone replacement therapy (Nordin et al, 1980), calcium, vitamin D, anabolic steroids (Chestnut et al, 1981), fluoride

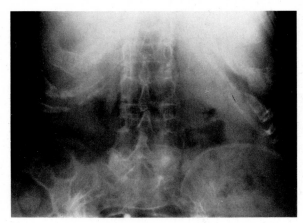

Fig. 20.5   An antero posterior radiograph of a 74 year old woman with osteoporosis. There is impingement of the spinous processes from lumbar lordosis and loss of vertebral height. The left 12th rib was producing impingement pain on the iliac crest and this was relieved by rib excision.

(Riggs et al, 1982) and calcitonin (Stevenson et al, 1982, and Rico and Espinos, 1982), but it has yet to be proved that they can reduce the incidence of subsequent fractures. Perhaps as we improve our techniques of quantitating osteoporosis, we shall be better able to monitor the methods of its prevention, and eventually reduce a troublesome cause of back pain in the elderly.

REFERENCES

Adams M A, Hutton W C 1982 Prolapsed intervertebral disc, a hyperflexion injury. Spine 7: 184–191

Chesnut 111 C H, Baylink D J, Roos B A et al 1981 Hormonal control of calcium metabolism. Amsterdam: Exerpta Medica, 1, 247–255

Fin Biering Sorensen 1982 Low back trouble in a general population of 30–40–50 and 60 year old men and women. Danish Medical Bulletin 29: 289–299

Holdsworth F W 1963 Fractures dislocations and fracture-dislocations of the spine. Journal of Bone and Joint Surgery 45-B: 6–20

Langton C McD, Palmer S B, Porter R W 1984 Measurement of broad band ultrasonic attenuation in cancellous bone. Engineering in Medicine 13: 89–91

Nicoll E A 1949 Fractures of the dorso-lumbar spine. Journal of Bone and Joint Surgery 31-B: 376–394

Nordin B E C, Peacock M, Aaeon J et al 1980 Clinics in Endocrinology and Metabolism 9 (1): 177–205

Nordin B E C 1983 Osteoporosis. Bone and joint disease in the elderly. Wright V (ed) Churchill Livingstone, Edinburgh, London, Melbourne and New York. 167–180

Resnick D L 1982 Fish vertebrae. Arthritis and Rheumatism 25; 1073–1077

Rico H, Espinos D 1982 Personal experience in the treatment of postmenopausal osteoporosis. Medical Clinics (Barcelona) 78: 322–325

Riggs B L, Seeman E, Hodgson S F, Taves D R, O'Fallon W M 1982 Effect of the fluoride–calcium regimen on vertebral fracture occurrence in post-menopausal osteoporosis. New England Journal of Medicine 306: 446–450

Stevenson J C, Whitehead M I 1982 Postmenopausal osteoporosis. British Medical Journal 285: 585–588

Stevenson J C, White M C, Joplin G F, MacIntyre I 1982 Osteoporosis and Calcitonin deficiency. British Medical Journal 285: 1010–1011

Young M H 1973 Long term consequences of stable fractures of the thoracoci and lumbar vertebral bodies. Journal of Bone and Joint Surgery 55-B: 295–300

21

Repeat spinal surgery

Some of the failures of previous spinal surgery are amongst the most disabled of back sufferers (O'Brien, 1983). Our natural response is to consider helping them with a further operation, but if the results of spinal surgery are uncertain, undoubtably repeat surgery is much more unpredictable (Connelly, 1983). It should be approached with caution. The most recalcitrant pain problem is that associated with the multiple operated back.

WHEN WE ARE APPROACHED BY A PATIENT ASKING ABOUT THE VALUE OF A FURTHER SPINAL OPERATION, THERE ARE SEVERAL POSSIBILITIES TO CONSIDER

1. Was the first operation a failure because of a wrong diagnosis?
2. Was the first operation a failure because the diagnosis was correct but the operation was wrong?
3. Was the first operation a failure because even though the diagnosis of the organic problem was correct, and the operation correct, the patient assessment was inadequate?
4. Was the operation successful, but secondary pathology has developed producing a new genuine organic problem for which a new surgical remedy is worth considering?
5. Was the operation successful, but a new largely non organic element has developed causing considerable distress to the patient?

In order to resolve the problem, the patient needs a great deal of our time. The correct decisions are most likely to be made by a multi-disciplinary team approach. Where do we start? An accurate past history is essential, relying not upon the patient's memory, but upon all the available records from previous hospitals and from general practitioner notes. The memory is often clouded by grievances about litigation. Previous operative failure confuses the record, and history prior to an accident is forgotten. Waddell et al (1979) showed that compensation has a significant negative influence on the results of surgery for lumbar disc disease. In a study of Philadelphia firemen having surgery for a herniated lumbar disc, only one in thirteen had returned to work after one year (Menkowitz and Whittaker 1975).

An estimate of the severity of the present problem is measured not only by listening to the patient but by interviewing the spouse and talking to the general practitioner. An objective measure of the abnormal signs may need to be documented longitudinally. Hospital admission makes this possible, when the patient's activity and behaviour can be assessed by the physiotherapist, and drug requirements monitored by the nurses.

Few surgeons relish re-exploration without hard clinical and radiolical evidence. No investigation should be ignored that might help to determine the pain source and repeat radiculography, discography and CT scan may be necessary. There is no place for an exploratory operation.

CT provides unique evidence about the extent of previous surgery and demonstrates the shape and size of the vertebral canal. Epidural fibrosis is seen in 75 per cent of post-operative studies (Teplick and Haskin, 1983), but it is not easy to differentiate it from overlooked previous disc material.

A detailed psychological assessment is essential. An abnormal profile on the MMPI does not mean that repeat surgery will fail, but it directs the surgeon to factors other than the spine that may be responsible for back pain. There is no clear evidence that the

MMPI low back scale will differentiate between patients who will have a poor, fair or good outcome from spinal fusion (Wilfling et al, 1973). Neither does it appear to help to identify the non-organic from the organic back pain patients (Tsushima and Towne, 1979). Patients with a high hypochondriasis score generally have a poor outcome to treatment, but this is only one of many factors to be considered when contemplating repeat surgery.

Only when all the available evidence is assembled, will a conference between the many disciplines produce the best decision.

In practice, this time consuming, laborious approach to repeat surgery is rarely followed outside a few centres of excellence, but the failures that accompany hastily conceived operations, the time involved in attempting to repair the results of failures, and the distress caused to the patient, should make us pause before we recommend repeat spinal surgery. Rather than operate in desperation, we do well to recall the inverted proverb 'if at first you don't succeed, give up.'

1.   Case report — Wrong diagnosis

Mrs. J.M., a 53-year old housewife, had severe constant burning pain in the left leg from the buttock into the posterior thigh, behind the knee to the calf and ankle. It kept her awake at night and drove her husband and the local doctor to despair. She had had treatment for a root entrapment syndrome, first epidural injections, and eventually a decompression of the left L.5 root canal where degenerative change had been encroaching from the apophyseal joints. The operation had relieved symptoms for a short time. Whilst in the hospital, the nurses had observed that she was fairly comfortable until her husband arrived to visit her, and then she requested analgesics. She was referred to a pain clinic, and several pain-relieving techniques offered to her, but she was no better. On reviewing the details of the first operation, she had never had a radiculogram. This was performed and demonstrated a large meningioma at the level of L.3. It was removed and she lost her pain.

Surgery may fail because the diagnosis is right but the operation incorrect. A disc protrusion may have been identified radiologically but the wrong level approached by operating too high by failing to identify the sacrum. At times the wrong side is explored when a pre-operative skin mark would have prevented the mistake.

A disc protrusion may have been correctly diagnosed in the older patient and excised with poor results because stenosis and/or instability were not recognised as associated factors.

2.   Case report — Wrong operation

Mr. J.K., a 47-year-old lorry driver, attended with pain in his back and root pain down to the left foot. Three years ago he had had a disc removed without much success. The previous hospital notes suggested that he had had surgery for pain in the back and left thigh. Straight leg raising had been 80/80 and there were no abnormal neurological signs. The lateral view of a radiculogram had shown a disc protrusion at L.4/5 but there was no cut-off of the nerve root dural sheath. The disc protrusion had been excised, but with no relief of symptoms. Once on his feet, his pain recurred.

A new radiograph showed further narrowing at L.4/5 disc space. Posterior indentation of the dural column remained on the radiculogram much as three years before, and a CT scan identified a very shallow vertebral canal at L.5 (1.2 cm). Originally he had certainly had symptoms related to a disc protrusion where there was probably some unnatural segmental movement. We would not expect such a combination of factors to be helped by removing the disc protrusion alone. A decompression would have had more chance of success, possibly without incising the annulus of the disc.

3. Case report — inadequate patient assessment

Mr. P.T. said he first hurt his back lifting at work, quickly developed pain down the right leg, and was admitted for bed rest. He failed to respond and was given a plaster jacket, which he found uncomfortable. The surgeon was reluctant to operate because although the symptoms remained, there were some signs of exaggeration. A neurologist confirmed the opinion that the symptoms were not all related to an organic problem, but the patient found his way to a further surgeon who performed a radiculogram. It demonstrated a small disc protrusion at L.4/5 level. This was removed through a fenestration, but the patient was no better. He says he is in constant pain; he walks with a stick and is seeking recompense for a disabling industrial accident.

4.   Case Report — Recurrence of back pain after successful surgery,? iatrogenic

Mrs. F.W. had an L.4/5 disc sequestration removed through a fenestration at 32 years of age, and had twelve good years without any back symptoms. She then presented with left L.5 root pain from the buttock, thigh to the calf, with pins and needles in the big toe. It was fairly constant, worse sitting for long and walking far. Straight leg raising was 90/80 and there were no abnormal neurological signs. She had some reduction of the L.4/5 disc space with osteophyte formation of the vertebral margins. A radiculogram was normal. She was given two epidural injections which provided only temporary relief, and because of continuing pain over an eighteen month period, she requested further surgery. A CT scan confirmed a shallow central canal at L.5, trefoil in shape. At operation, there was a posterior vertebral bar on the lower border of L.4 and upper border of L.5 with a tough ridged annulus, to which the thickened L.5 root was closely apposed. The laminae of L.5 and half of L.4 were removed, decompressing the shallow trefoil canal, and the L.5 root followed well into the root canal. There was a slow improvement with reduction in the degree of root pain over twelve months, but she still admits to some intermittent root pain.

Case report

Mrs. G.E. at 34 years of age had several pieces of disc material removed which had extruded deep to the posterior longitudinal ligament at L.5/S.1 on the left, relieving L.5 root symptoms. S.L.R. had been 70/40 and she quickly returned to a normal active painfree life. Two years later she developed pain in the opposite thigh which spread to the calf. It varied in severity, sometimes putting her to bed for days at a time. Two epidural injections gave temporary relief but she began taking large doses of analgesics and tranquilisers. She listed to the left, was a little tender at L.5, had S.L.R. 70/90, and a CT scan showed an overhanging superior facet at S.1 on the right with probable disc material anterior to the L.5 root, (Fig. 21.1). The root was decompressed surgically by undercutting the facet and after incising the anulus anterior to the root, a large sequestrated piece of disc material was removed. This was either symptomless from the first operation or was 'fresh herniation' of nucleus.

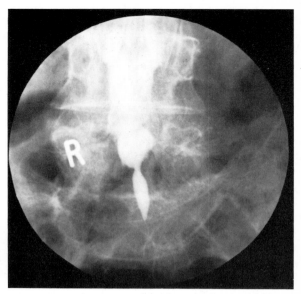

Fig. 21.2 A radiculogram of a patient with 'arachnoiditis', occlusion of the root sheaths and tapering of the metrizamide column after a previous decompressive laminectomy.

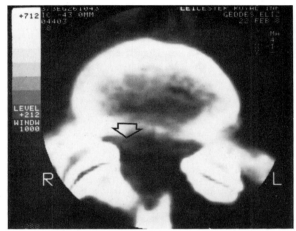

Fig. 21.1 CT scan of L.5 showing a disc protrusion on the right with an overhanging superior facet compromising the L.5 root.

Post operative arachnoiditis and extradural fibrosis

The cause of failed spinal surgery when a patient has continuing back pain and discomfort in the legs for no apparent cause is often attributed to 'arachnoiditis' — an inflammatory process leading to fibrosis, which binds together the roots of the cauda equina. It is probably over-diagnosed. A repeat myelogram may show concentric narrowing of the terminal theca with occlusion of the root sheaths and tapering of the metrizamide column (Fig. 21.2) and the term 'arachnoiditis' becomes a convenient diagnosis. Because we do not perform myelography on symptomless post operative patients, we do not know if these radiological appearances are the inevitable consequence of surgery for many healthy patients.

The appearance of arachnoiditis at operation, however, is not in question. The dura appears white instead of blue, it is opaque rather than translucent, and its contents firm and resistant to pressure. A small incision into the dura will fail to produce a bead of cerebro-spinal fluid, but rather the dura and underlying arachnoid is adherent in a mass of fibrous tissue.

Arachnoiditis produces aching and burning pain in the lower back, buttocks and perineum, but pain in a root distribution, although it may co-exist, is probably from other causes. Extra-dural scarring often accompanies arachnoiditis, which will limit the normal excursion of the nerve roots. Associated bony or soft tissue encroachment into the root canal adds to the problem and produces root symptoms.

We know neither the cause nor the remedy for arachnoiditis. Extradural fibrosis can be reduced by the application of a fat graft over the dura at the time of operation. This is probably unnecessary if only a small area of dura is exposed, such as when removing a disc protrusion through a fenestration, but with a larger area of decompression, it is worth applying a prophylactic fat graft. This can be obtained from the subcutaneous tissues at the site of incision in women, and many male patients, but a separate buttock incision may be necessary for donor fat in the less obese male.

The principals of skin grafting apply to fat grafts.

Vascularisation depends on peripheral ingrowth of vessels and firm apposition to the recipient bed. A large volume of fat with small surface area is less likely to survive than a smaller volume with larger surface area. Thin postage stamp size grafts of 5 millimeters thickness are probably ideal. If the graft is floating in a haematoma it is less likely to vascularise than a graft seated between the dura and paraspinal muscles. A loose deep muscle suture helps to reduce the dead space and vacuum drainage reduces the possibility of haematoma. Pedicle fat grafts are less successful than free grafts (Krempen and Silver 1984).

Arachnoiditis should not preclude further operation when attempting to treat the post-laminectomy back pain. If restriction of space within the vertebral canal is an associated factor, then good results can be expected from decompression if it is sufficiently radical (Parke et al, 1981). If, however, the symptoms are related to instability, decompression can only compound the problem. O'Brien (1983) has some success from combined anterior and posterior fusion for selected post-laminectomy back pain patients, suggesting that for some, instability is a significant factor.

5.   Case report — successful story — subsequent distress

Mr. H.W., now 62 years of age, can walk only 200 yards before he stops with tired legs. Twenty years ago he had a disc removed, and worked consistently at a light job until 5 years ago. He became unemployed and thinks his legs started to ache at that time. Does he have neurogenic claudication requiring canal decompression?

He complains not only of the legs and back, but of the thoracic spine and anginal pain. Previous depressive illness has made him seek psychiatric help. He exhibits several inappropriate clinical signs, has good peripheral pulses, and a radiculogram although suggesting some distal arachnoiditis, confirms an adequate canal above L.5. There is so much evidence of distress, that although there may well be an organic element to his back symptoms, further spinal surgery is likely to add to his back symptoms.

Repeat spinal surgery can be rewarding, but should be approached with great care. There are too many patients who have followed a disastrous trail, first a disc operation then dissection of adhesions or spinal fusion, followed by further rhizolysis or correction of a failed fusion, and then a decompression, even rhizotomy or spinothalamic tractotomy. Before embarking on any spinal operation, we would do well to consider whether every reasonable conservative approach has been tried. Unsatisfactory surgical procedures produce far greater degrees of painful disability than does the unoperated lumbar spine.

REFERENCES

Connolly J F 1983 Does operative treatment of lumbar disc syndrome produce more disability than it prevents? The Nebraska Medical Journal, June 1983: 155–156
Krempen J F and Silver R 1984 Pedicle fat grafts is a method of preventing excess cicatrix formation following laminectomy: analysis of 103 cases. Presented to the International Society for the Study of the Lumbar Spine, Montreal
Menkowitz E, Whittaker R 1975 The Spine 2: 503
O'Brien J P 1983 The role of fusion for chronic low back pain. The Orthopaedic Clinics of North America 14: 639–647
Parke W W, Gammell K, Rothman R H 1981 Arterial vascularisation of the cauda equina. Journal of Bone and Joint Surgery 63–A: 53–61

Teplick J G, Haskin M E 1983 CT of the post-operative lumbar spine. Radiological Clinics of North America 21: 395–420
Tsushima W T, Towne W S 1979 Clinical limitations of the low back scale. Journal of Clinical Psychology 35: 306–308
Waddell G, Kummel E G, Lotto W N, Graham J D, Hall H, McCulloch J A 1979 Failed lumbar disc surgery and repeat surgery following industrial injuries. Journal of Bone and Joint Surgery 61–A: 201–207
Wilfling F J, Klonoff H, Kokan P 1973 Psychological, demographic and orthopaedic factors associated with prediction of outcome of spinal fusion. Clinical Orthopaedics and Related Research 90: 153–160

22

Back pain — an exhibition of distress

We have previously discussed ways of recognising patients whose behaviour appears to be disproportionate to the organic spinal problem (page 54). The clinician begins to recognise these patients intuitively though Waddell et al (1980 and 1984) has encouraged a more systematic documentation of those spinal symptoms and signs that suggest exaggeration.

AETIOLOGY

For the majority of patients, exaggeration is an unconscious response to one or several motivating causes. Fear of cancer, fear of a crippling illness, fear of paralysis may initiate a neurological process that results in exaggeration. The same process may develop from a desire to gain, whether it be financially by litigation, socially by not having to continue in an unpleasant occupation, or domestically by receiving the sympathy of family and friends. Other emotions may trigger the same response. Aggression and a desire for vengeance on the employer, the medical profession, or the spouse, may stimulate the same exaggeration.

There is much evidence that this exaggerated reaction to a relatively less significant organic spinal problem is constitutionally or environmentally predetermined from an early age, though a life changing event may be the precipitating cause of symptoms, (Leavitt et al 1979, Higgs, 1984). Letham et al, (1983) have shown that individuals in early adult life tend to react in the same way to any external pain source, some making much of it, and others little. Petrie (1978) has shown that some individuals are 'enhancers' of pain, whilst others are 'reducers', a characteristic that is reflected in other life attitudes. Psychological studies of patients with chronic back pain, show that some subjects with low extraversion, high neuroticism and high somatisation, suffer greatly. (Hanvik, 1966, Sternback et al, 1973, Marute et al, 1976). It suggests that personality predetermines the way in which a patient will respond to a mechanical disturbance of the spine. How much of this is genetically determined, and how much related to environment has yet to be resolved. Patients attending a general practitioner with back pain are no more likely to have psychological or psychiatric problems than other patients (Gilchrist, 1983), but when assessing the relatively few patients with chronic back pain, there does seem to be a high proportion with psychological and psychotic disturbance (Lloyd et al, 1979). Psychosocial problems can prolong the course of physical illness and lead to chronic invalidism.

The clinician who is first consulted about back pain, bears a great responsibility for the subsequent behaviour of that patient. If he fails to recognise the potential for abnormal pain behaviour, he may unwittingly enhance fears by over-investigation, unnecessary treatment, and prolonged rest, when confident encouragement to graduated increasing activity may be in the patient's interest.

We are still appallingly ignorant about abnormal illness behaviour. We can recognise it, postulate about causative mechanisms, but we know nothing of the neurological mechanism, and whether we are dealing with one problem varying in degree, or several conditions. It is not surprising that our attempts to modify it usually fail (McCreary et al, 1979).

Exaggeration may, of course, be a conscious deliberate attempt to deceive, but this probably represents only a small proportion of exaggerating patients.

RECOGNITION OF DISTRESS

One of the benefits of clinical maturity is a growing ability to recognise the patient whose distress outweighs the recognisable organic pathology. One is constantly alert for mistakes, and the possibility of overlooking a treatable lesion, but intuitively it becomes possible to recognise those patients with an exaggerated response, (Fig. 22.1). Their facial expression, the adjectives they use for pain, and the inappropriate signs (page 55) suggest distress. We recognise psychiatric disturbances in the unco-operative, noisy, weepy, agitated patient, but this is often hidden in the quiet and uncomplaining, (Nabarro 1984). Ransford et al, (1976) have popularised the use of 'pain drawings' which can be

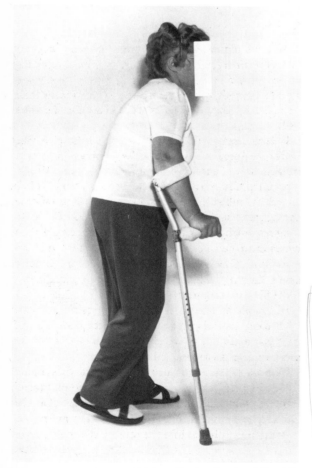

Fig. 22.1 A patient complaining of back pain who walks with elbow crutches either has a serious neurological problem or is exhibiting signs of distress.

assessed at a glance, and avoid the need for a complicated scoring system. This subjective documentation is said to correlated well with hypochondriasis and hysteria. It is not recognition of abnormal pain behaviour, but its modification that is difficult.

MANAGEMENT

We are singularly unsuccessful in our efforts to help the patient with abnormal illness behaviour. It is a source of disappointment that we are least able to help those patients with the most intense suffering.

We cannot detect much organic pathology (though it does not mean that it is not there), and generally our therapeutic efforts fail to reduce the level of distress. Failure to respond to treatment is, in fact, one inappropriate symptom. If we try to identify a motivating cause such as fear, attempts to reassure are often unrewarding. It is sometimes suggested that when litigation has been settled, and the gainful motive is no longer necessary, symptoms will resolve (Miller, 1961), but this is rarely true. Although it is essential to be sure that there is no treatable organic problem that has caused exaggerated pain behaviour, negative invasive investigations sometimes actually increase the morbidity, (Herkowitz et al 1983). All too often a myelogram does not show pathology and the procedure increases the anxiety level of the patient. This must be weighed against ignoring a possible spinal tumour.

Some patients with back pain benefit from a team approach (Bartorelli, 1983), and probably none more than the distressed patient. A psychiatric and psychological assessment is time consuming but helpful. If often explains the distress if it cannot change it. We have had a little success using the methods of Roberts and Reinhardt (1980) attempting to modify behaviour. When a patient shows gross signs of exaggeration, provided there is no significant organic problem that requires treatment, and no psychiatric disorder, they are offered a programme of non-reward for abnormal behaviour. Patients are excluded if they are seeking compensation, and they must accept the objectives and methods of the programme.

They and their spouse attend a multi-disciplinary conference with their general practitioner, orthopaedic surgeon, pain specialist, psychologist, physiotherapist and pharmacist. If accepted for the programme, they are asked to agree to defined objectives, such as withdrawal from all analgesic drugs, removing walking aids, correcting abnormal posture, performing household chores, gardening, improving social contacts, developing hobbies, recreations, even returning to work. The relief or reduction of pain is not included in the objectives.

Increasing activity in spite of pain, may in fact reduce the level of suffering. B-endorphins and meta-encephalins are released with treadmill exercise (Howlett et al 1984), and by encouraging a more energetic lifestyle, we may increase the release of these endogenous opioid peptides.

Over a three week period the patient is seen daily as an out-patient in the physiotherapy department. Abnormal behaviour is actively discouraged, and acceptable behaviour commended. They are commended for walking without aids, for correct posture, but reprimanded for unacceptable behaviour. The spouse takes the same attitude at home, being unsympathetic to any pain responses, and a diary for the patient and spouse helps to confirm compliance, (Petty and Mastria, 1983). The general practitioner likewise refrains from a supporting attitude to pain. A cocktail of the patient's analgesic drugs is administered with decreasing concentration until there are no active ingredients at all.

After three weeks some patients surprise themselves by their achievements, discarding their therapeutic and walking aids, and living more purposeful lives. Not all are successful.

The pain clinic

Our understanding of pain is still in its infancy, but it is encouraging that clinicians and particularly anaesthetists, are attempting to grapple with the problem of pain (Bonica, 1976 and Lancet, 1982). The development of Pain Clinics where the many techniques that reduce pain sensation can be offered to the chronic back pain sufferer is helpful to both patient and doctor alike.

Not all of the methods used in a pain clinic are of proven value, but many patients are referred because they experience severe pain for which no remedy has been found, and they are grateful that someone is still prepared to try.

1. Who is referred?

It is important that patients attending a Pain Clinic have been fully investigated to ensure that there is no hidden pathology remedial to treatment. They are patients who have usually been told that there is no surgical remedy to their problem. The possible source of pain has been explained, with an attempt to allay unreasonable fears. They have attended the 'Back School' and know how to live with their pain, how to minimise spinal stress and accept their disability, and yet the pain remains and they are still unsatisfied. These patients can find the pain clinic invaluable.

2. What can be offered?

If the methods of treatment are unproven, we may question their value. However, to the individual patient there is no doubt that a caring physician, attempting to help a patient come to terms with their pain, is the answer to their problems, for the time being at least.

It is necessary to make a careful appraisal of the drug regime, especially the analgesics, anti inflammatory, anti-depressants and hypnotic drugs. Too often drugs have become habit-forming. They are producing side effects and have lost their efficacy by aggravating the symptoms (Sternbach, 1970). Unquestionably many patients with abnormal pain behaviour receive excessive medication and reduction is difficult. The anaesthetist is probably best fitted to assess the drug requirements, which probably varies for different categories of pain.

Injections of trigger points and fibrositic nodules, with local anaesthetic and steroid can give relief of pain for a time. Superficial injection into a tender sacro iliac area can be similarly helpful.

The apophyseal joint can be investigated as a pain source by placing a needle under radiographic control into the joint, and injecting local anaesthetic. If the clinician is confident that this identifies a pain source, he may inject phenol into the joint. Other methods of capsular denervation include radio-frequency block, (Mehta and Sluijter, 1979).

The critics of these methods remind us of the problems. It is difficult to be sure of needle placement into a small spinal joint. Local anaesthetic will diffuse widely from the joint into the root canal, and into the surrounding soft tissues making interpretation of pain relief difficult. And denervation of a joint can produce a Charcot's joint, with possible future problems.

There are, however, inumerable enthusiasts convinced that apophyseal joint injections are of value. If so many patients are relieved by such a simple manoeuvre, the surgeon must ask himself whether some of his operative successes are also the result of denervation. Those who practise radiofrequency facet denervation claim to have encouraging results provided patients are carefully selected, and properly managed (Rashbaum, 1983 and Oudehoven, 1979). It is suggested that some patients experience pain in the back, referred into the thigh or upper calf, from noxious stimulation of the posterior primary ramus supplying the apophyseal joints. Such pain is said to be worse with activity, such as twisting and bending, and is relieved by rest. Signs are few, except that torsion of the spine causes pain, and the affected segment is tender to pressure. It is difficult, of course, to confirm that these criteria represent a pain source just because a facet injection into the joint relieves pain temporarily, or because a facet block to the triple innervation of the joint gives pain relief. The protagonists, however, claim at least a 70 per cent success rate with radiofrequency facet denervation under general anaesthetic, provided a facet injection and block relieve much of the pre-injection pain. No doubt there are many satisfied patients and some pain clinics do find this a useful technique for chronic back pain.

Epidural injections, if carefully performed, are relatively innocuous and often helpful. We have restricted their use to patients with root entrapment and post operative patients with continuing back or leg pain. It may have a wider role.

Clinicians have often found it difficult to know whether to recommend acupuncture when all other treatments for chronic back pain have failed. Trials that will convince the sceptics are very hard to design (Lewith 1984). Some reports have been encouraging (Sato and Nakatani, 1974, and Sechzer and Leung, 1974 and Lewit 1979). Two controlled double blind trials suggested that acupuncture can be superior to placebo (Matsumoto et al, 1974 and Man and Baragar, 1974). On the other hand, five trials found no difference (Lee et al, 1975, Gaw et al, 1975, Moore and Berk, 1976, Edelist et al, 1976, and Mendelson et al, 1983). The counter irritant effect of stimulating the skin in a noxious manner with subcutaneous acupuncture needles was found to be superior to placebo dummy surface electrodes on both subjective and objective assessment of back pain by Macdonald et al, 1983. The evaluation of acupuncture trials is extremely difficult (Lewith and Machin, 1983), but irrespective of trials, some patients find relief from the technique.

The relief of pain by counter irritation is an extension of the common practice of rubbing a painful area. The application of superficial counter irritant was shown to be useful by Melzack et al (1977) and Simons (1975) and many patients find useful painful relief from using transcutaneous nerve stimulation, (Miles, 1984).

3. Assessment

A major problem in deciding the effectiveness of treatment for back pain, is the difficulty in assessing outcome, especially when the difference in improvement between two groups of patients is relatively small. Disability may be measured by asking the patient to record their own subjective disability, or by a doctor's more objective criteria. There may be a difference between the two (Dunt et al, 1980) and some would argue that self-rated assessment, though prone to subjective error, can be more sensitive (Roland et al, 1983). Time drags for the patient in pain, and assessment of time, may be useful pain related parameter (Bilting et al 1983). Measuring success is important and this opportunity is not lost in many pain clinics, (Lancet 1982). In spite of the difficulty in assessing the value of many of the old and new remedies, perhaps the most useful development of the pain clinic is the opportunity it gives to support a distressed patient at a time of crisis.

REFERENCES

Bartorelli D 1983 Low back pain: a team approach. Journal of Neurosurgery 15: 41–44

Bilting M, Carlsson C, Menge B, Pellettieri L and Peterson L 1983. Estimation of time as a measure of pain magnitude. Journal of Psychosomatic Research. 27: 493–497

Bonica J J 1976 The introduction to the first world congress of Pain. Goals of the IASP and the world congress: Advances in Pain Research and Therapy Vol: 1, New York, Raven Press, 26–39

Dunt D R, Kaufert J M, Corkhill R et al 1980 A technique for precisely measuring activities of daily living. Community Medicine 2: 120–125

Edelist G, Gross A E, Langer F 1976 Treatment of low back pain with acupuncture Can Anaesth Soc. J.23: 303–306

Gaw A C, Chang L W, Shaw L C 1975 Efficiency of acupuncture on osteoarthritic pain. New England Journal Medicine 293: 375–378

Gilchrist I C 1983 Psychological aspects of acute low back pain in general practice. Journal of Royal College of General Practitioners 33: 417–419

Hanvik L J 1966 MMPI profiles in patients with low back pain. Basic Readings on the MMPI in Psychology and Medicine Welsh GS,, Dahlstrom WG (eds) Minneapolis: University of Minnesota Press

Herkowitz H N, Romeyn R L, Rothman R H 1983 The indications for metrizamide myelography. Journal of Bone and Joint Surgery 65-A: 1144–1149

Higgs R 1984 Life changes. British Medical Journal 288: 1556–1557

Howlett T A, Tomlin S, Ngahfoong L, Rees L H, Bullen B A, Skrinar G S and McArthur J W 1984 Release of B endorphin and met-enkephalin during exercise in normal women: response to training. British Medical Journal 288: 1950–1952

Lancet editorial 1982. Lancet 1: 486–487

Leavitt F, Garron D C, D'Angelo C M and McNeill T W 1979 Low back pain in patients with and without demonstrable organic disease. Pain 6: 191–200

Lee P K, Andersen T W, Modell J H, Saga S A 1975 Treatment of chronic pain with acupuncture. JAMA 232: 1133–1135

Letham J, Slade P D, Troup J D G, Bentley G 1983 Outline of a fear-avoidance model of exaggerated pain perception. Behaviour Research Therapy 21: 401–408

Lewit K 1979 The needle effect in the relief of myofascial pain. Pain 6: 83–90

Lewith G T, Machin D 1983 The evaluation of the clinical effects of acupuncture. Pain 16: 111–127

Lewith G T 1984 Can we assess the effects of acupuncture? British Medical Journal 288: 1475–1476

Lloyd G G, Wolkind S N, Greenwood R, Harris D J 1979 A psychiatric study of patients with persistent low back pain. Rheumatology and Rehabilitation 18: 30–34

McCreary C, Turner J, Dawson E 1979 The MMPI as a predictor of response to conservative treatment for low back pain. Journal of Clinical Psychology 35: 278–284

Macdonald A J R, Macrae K D, Master B R, Rubin A P 1983 Superficial acupuncture in the relief of chronic low back pain. Annals of the Royal College of Surgeons of England 65: 44–46

Man S C, Baragar F D 1974 Preliminary clinical study of acupuncture in rheumatoid arthritis. Journal of Rheumatology 1: 126–129

Maruta T, Swansoin D W, Swenson W M 1976 Pain as a psychiatric symptom: Comparison between low back pain and depression. Psychosomatics 17: 123–127

Matsumoto T, Levy B, Ambrus O V 1974 Clinical evaluation of acupuncture. Am Surg. 40: 400–405

Mehta M, Sluijter M E 1979 The treatment of chronic pain. A preliminary survey of the effect of radiofrequency denervation of the posterior vertebral joints. Anaesthesia 34: 768

Melzack R, Stillwell D M, Fox E J 1977 Trigger points and acupuncture points for pain: correlations and implications. Pain 3: 3–23

Mendelson G, Selwood T S, Kranz H, Kidson M A, Scott D S 1983 Acupuncture treatment for chronic back pain: a double blind placebo-controlled trial. The American Journal of Medicine 74: 49–55

Miles J 1984 Electrical stimulation for the relief of pain. Annals of the Royal College of Surgeons of England 66: 108–112

Miller H 1961 Accident neurosis. British Medical Journal 1961: i: 919–925

Moore M E, Berk S N 1976 Acupuncture for chronic shoulder pain. Ann. Intern Med. 84: 381–384

Nabarro J 1984 Unrecognised psychiatric illness in medical patients. British Medical Journal 289: 635–636

Oudehoven R C 1979 The role of laminectomy, facet rhizotomy and epidural steroids. Spine 4: 145–147

Petrie A 1978 Individuality in pain and suffering. Second edition. The University of Chicago Press, Chicago, London

Petty N E, Mastria M A 1983 Management of compliance to progressive relaxation and orthopaedic exercises in treatment of chronic back pain. Psychological Reports 52: 35–38

Ransford A O, Cairns D, Mooney V 1976 The pain drawing as an aid to the psychogenic evaluation of patients with low back pain. Spine 1: 127–134

Rashbaum R F 1983 Radiofrequency facet denervation: a treatment alternative in refractory low back pain with or without leg pain. The Orthopaedic Clinics or North America 14: 569–575

Roberts A H, Reinhardt L 1980 The behavioural management of chronic pain: Long term follow up with comparison groups. Pain 8: 151–162

Roland M O, Morrell D C, Morris R W 1983 Can general practitioners predict the outcome of episodes of back pain? British Medical Journal 286: 523–525

Sato N, Nakatani Y 1974 Acupuncture for chronic pain in Japan. Adv. Neurology 4: 813–818

Sechzer P H 1975 Acupuncture: Surgical aspects. Bull NY Acad Med 51: 922–929

Simons D G 1975 Muscle pain syndromes. Part 1 American Journal Physical Medicine 54: 289–311

Sternbach R A, Wolf S R, Murphy R W 1973 Aspects of Chronic low back pain. Psychosomatics 18: 52–56

Sternbach R A 1970 Strategies and tactics in the treatment of patients with pain in B L Crue (ed) Pain and Suffering: Selected Aspects. C C Thomas

Waddell G, McCulloch J A, Kummell E and Venner R M 1980 Nonorganic physical signs in low back pain. Spine 5: 117–125

Waddell G, Main C J, Morris E W, Di Paola M and Gray I C M 1984 Chronic low back pain, psychological distress and illness behaviour. Spine 9: 209–213

23

Prevention of back pain

Statistics from my own hospital two centuries ago showed a remarkable rate of cure (Fig. 23.1). Could we do but the same today. Perhaps we are more aware of our failures. Our traditional remedies for low back pain are being exposed in the light of scientific assessment, with what shattering results. Treatments that we have accepted from circumstantial evidence have been proved ineffective, little better than doing nothing at all.

INADEQUACY OF CONVENTIONAL TREATMENT

Part of the problem in assessing treatment lies in diagnosis (Morrison, 1983). One would not expect impressive results if a particular remedy is offered to all types of back pain. In addition, we need better methodology in trials, blindness of therapy, measurement of compliance and careful assessment of outcome to prove that a treatment for a particular back pain syndrome is effective (Deyo, 1983). Until such information is available, we are bound to regard many of our longstanding therapies with suspicion.

Doran and Newell (1975) and Coxhead et al (1981) compared traction, exercises, manipulation and corsets in multicentric trials. They did not show that any one method was better than another, except that in the short term several treatments with active physiotherapy had value. Edwards (1969) and Lewith and Turner (1982) likewise thought that manipulation could get their general practice patients back to work sooner, but admitted inadequacies in their studies. In the long term, randomised mobilisation and manipulation of the lumbar spine is ineffective for back pain (Sims-Williams et al, 1978), and intermittent traction does little for disc prolapse (Weber, 1973). Maitland mobilisation is effective above the lower lumbar level when pain tenderness and limited movement is believed to be related to the apophyseal joints.

Spinal manipulation and mobilisation of the lumbar spine has long been used around the world with success. Unfortunately there is no scientific proof that it works, why it works and for what conditions it works best. McKenzie (1981) has tried to define pain patterns and postures that will respond to manipulation and self mobilisation techniques. My own view is that until there is better evidence that patients with defined back pain syndromes can benefit from manipulative or other physiotherapy

THE PRESENT STATE OF DONCASTER.

The report of patients taken in at the Dispensary from Oct. 1, 1792, to Oct. 1, 1803.

Patients admitted - - - - - - - -	4885
Cured - - - - - - - - - - - - -	4295
Dead - - - - - - - - - - - -	209
Relieved - - - - - - - - - - -	234
Incurable - - - - - - - - - -	10
Irregular - - - - - - - - - - -	50
Remaining on the books - - - -	87

Fig. 23.1 Hospital statistics for the Doncaster dispensary in 1803.

treatment, for many patients the time is more profitably spent talking with them, helping them manage this episode, and avoid the next.

How successful are our drugs? Analgesics are necessary for acute back pain, and for the sleepless patient, but for chronic back pain, placebo seems to be as effective as analgesic drugs (Berry et al, 1981). Tranquilisers and anti-inflammatory drugs are no better than analgesics for the acute disc lesion (Weber, 1980 and Weber and Aasand, 1980).

Corsets have been used for centuries and are manufactured in their thousands. Are they over prescribed? We cannot deny their value when so many find security in a lumbar support after the acute attack of pain, and the elderly return for more. There is a great lack of compliance, but is this success or failure? Success that the pain has settled with the corset and it is no longer needed? Or failure because it did not help?

When a corset eases pain, we do not know why. Is it the reduction of movement?

Fiddler (1983) showed that a canvas corset reduced the angular movement of the lumbar spine by two-thirds, but there are times when it will actually increase movement at the lumbo-sacral junction, (Norton and Brown, 1957, Lumsden and Morris, 1968). A support within the corset gives better relief than the same canvas without support (Million et al, 1981). There are added factors of the corset increasing intra-abdominal pressure, providing relief by local warmth, and by stimulating mechano-receptors.

A corset should probably be reserved for the period of recovery after a severe acute episode of derangement, for a few weeks after a spinal fusion, and for the patient with longstanding instability symptoms. It is not the panacea for all backache.

Neither is surgery the answer to back pain. It is a last resort. The disappointing operative results are no greater than those of other disciplines, but because back pain does not kill and will rarely paralyse, most spinal surgeons are probably unique among their colleagues: they occupy their time finding ways of relieving pain and improving function by non-operative means.

If patients can be steered into a programme of education, caring for their own back, trying to avoid future trouble, this is sometimes better than over enthusiastic remedies of untried worth.

PREVENTION

Because we so often fail to find a cure, there has been a strong swing of medical opinion towards prevention, seeking ways to avoid the first attack, ways to prevent spinal stress that hinders the natural healing of the present pain source, and to prevent the next episode. How can it be done? There are but three ways:

1. Altering the environment.
2. Altering the individual, changing attitudes and the use of the spine.
3. Identifying the individual at greatest risk and deploying him to work of lesser risk.

Ergonomics, education and screening.

1. Ergonomics

Ergonomics attempts to match the demands of the work to the ability of the worker, by modifying the working environment. Employers, if they would consider it, and employees if they knew it, have equal opportunity to ensure a safe working environment. There is broad agreement about what is unsafe for a spine. Posture is important. Lifting is often the final insult with its three variables, the weight of the object, how it is lifted and how often. Avoidance of accidents comes a close third.

Unacceptably high static spinal loads can develop when standing or sitting for long in the stooped posture, probably affecting disc nutrition and producing spinal muscle fatigue. At such a time the disc will be vulnerable to injury from inadvisable lifting. Modification of the working environment to provide a more acceptable working posture should reduce the incidence of back pain.

Attempts have been made to evaluate certain working activities, postures and spinal stresses, by measuring intradiscal pressure (Nachemson & Elfstrom, 1970), intra-abdominal pressure, electromyography (Schultz et al, 1982), and time spent in the flexed posture by using inclinometers. These techniques need further assessment and comparison before they can be meaningfully used in the working environment to measure spinal stress. Changing from the supine to the erect stooped posture increases the intradiscal pressure six fold (Nachemson and Elfstrom, 1970), and patterns of lifting correlate with intra-abdominal pressure (Davis and Stubbs, 1976 and 1977). By looking critically at working activities and postures that produce these high pressures, these can be modified to generate more acceptable spinal loads.

There is obviously a limit to the weight that can be safely lifted, but it is arbitrary. We probably have a built-in warning mechanism about weights that are too heavy, and trouble arises when a load is not properly assessed, when it is lifted without preparation. The working environment should allow for unacceptable loads to be lifted with assistance from colleagues or by mechanical aids, hoists, barrows and trolleys.

The manner of lifting is important, and if loads must be lifted at a distance from the body, either they should be reduced proportionally, or the method of lifting altered (Davis and Stubbs, 1977). Lifting can be made acceptable by altering the height and location of the working surface. Wearing suitable clothes for the job is important for the man afraid of getting his clean trousers dirty, or the nurse embarrassed and limited by stooping in a tight skirt. Safety training in industry has for many years emphasised the presumed advantage of lifting with the trunk erect, using the lower limb muscles to reduce the compressive load on the lumbar spine (Troup, 1977). There is no doubt that this requires a greater expenditure of energy, because there is a vertical displacement of a greater proportion of the body weight when lifting with bent knees. It is, however, thought to be less stressful on the lumbar spine. Leskinen et al (1983) have shown that the benefits of the leg lift are only superior to the back lift provided the weight is kept close to the body, and this is not always possible if the knees are bent. Advocates of kinetic lifting believe there is less spinal stress if the load is first pulled horizontally towards the body before being swung upwards (the load kinetic lift), or if the hips are first moved vertically before the load is lifted from the floor (the trunk kinetic lift), but this has yet to be proved. Perhaps the best advice to protect the lumbar spine is to lift from the bent knee position, having the load as close to the body's centre of gravity as possible, stoop slightly forwards with a lordotic spine and do most of the work with the legs. The initial major work is accomplished by the hip extensors. Watching a weight lifter can be informative (Fig. 23.2).

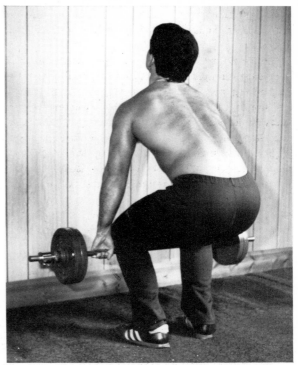

Fig. 23.2   The professional weight lifter lifts with flexed hips and knees and is stooped slightly forwards with a lordotic spine.

There is no doubt that a man with a healthy back can do more work and expend less energy by using a back lift with extended legs, but this is not a position to recommend if the spine is vulnerable.

Spinal structures are more subject to injury when fatigued, and the frequency of lifting must be considered in any job. Periods of rest can be productive.

It is not possible to estimate the importance of 'accidents' at work, because of the natural tendencies to associate a causative episode to the experience of pain. As many as a third of back pain episodes at work are recorded as truly accidental injuries (Troup, 1983). Many patients blame some injury like slipping, stumbling, falling or having something fall on them, with subsequent back pain, but the avoidance of accidents should be as much the responsibility of the employee as the employer. Although falls are not the major cause of accidental back pain, they do have a poor prognosis (Manning and Shannon, 1979, and Troup, 1981). Respect for the regulations, clean floor surfaces, care in performing the job is as important as adequate lighting, plenty of space and safe machinery. Anticipation is an essential part of avoiding back injury.

Some employers concerned about the incidence of back pain amongst their staff, are prepared to seek the help of ergonomists. They identify the areas of high and low incidence of back pain by documentation of every back injury and absenteeism due to back pain, and then study the working activities in the area of high risk. Sophisticated measuring apparatus may help (Otun et al, 1984) but this is not always necessary in order to recommend modifications.

There are, however, limitations to the application of ergonomic principles in real life. The mining industry is an example of excellent mechanisation on the surface, where in the stock yard, tons of equipment are moved with little or no manual handling. Underground, however, although the back-breaking pick and shovel belongs to another era, there are times when tons of face machinery must be manipulated into a confined coal face, and repaired when it fails. The fluid nature of the underground strata means constant damage to supports and machinery, which can only be corrected by physical spinal effort (Fig. 23.3).

The nurse is faced with the same dilemma (Scholey, 1983). Areas of high and low risk have been identified in hospitals. Orthopaedic and geriatric wards are more hazardous for the nurse's back than surgical wards and out patients' department (Lloyd et al, 1979). The relationship between back pain and patient handling and nurse status is conflicting (Stubbs et al, 1983). Nursing administrators now more aware of the risks, are obliged to provide lifting hoists for patients in hospital and at home. The height of beds, and nurses uniforms are planned with spinal safety in mind. But in spite of every care and effort to improve the environment, the unexpected can happen; a heavy patient moves awkwardly, the nurse slips, and an injury occurs.

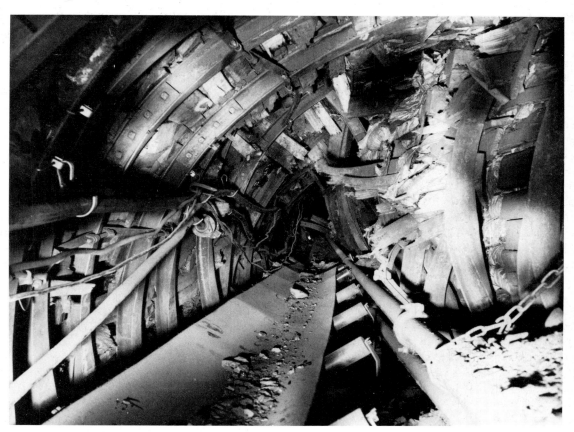

Fig. 23.3 Photograph of the fluid geological conditions of a coal mine.

2. Education

Education of the young

Every patient with a damaged disc would choose to turn the clock back and start with a healthy spine again, with a knowledge about its anatomy, physiology and limitations. But it is too late. They regret the abuse of earlier years, and wish someone had told them that there was a correct way to lift, and that a disc has limited strength.

We can only speculate at present whether there would be less back pain if the sufferers had been better informed before the first injury. Some could argue that if a disc is inherently weak, it will prolapse under normal stresses, and that education is superfluous. Even if it were of value, information may be quickly forgotten by those for whom back pain is not part of their experience. 'What I hear I forget, what I see I remember, what I do I know.' Education may even be counter-productive to concentrate on spinal pain in a neurotic society, of which back pain is but one symptom.

Others would suggest that all knowledge is valuable, and that with something as important as the human spine, it is unreasonable to withhold information about its structure and limited strength. Health education shares knowledge of diet, sex and addiction. Why should a healthy spine be excluded? If it is accepted that knowledge important to our well being should be shared, then the young deserve 'back education'.

1. Teachers of biology have an opportunity to teach spinal structure, function and limitations, in their syllabus. The lumbar spine is a prime example of the wedding between structure and function, but compared with other human systems, it receives a disproportionately smaller share of study. A healthy theoretical understanding of the spine, reinforced by its rightful place in an examination, may be remembered with benefit in later years, (Figs. 23.4, 23.5).

2. Teachers of physics already teach principles of levers, pressures and osmosis. An application of these

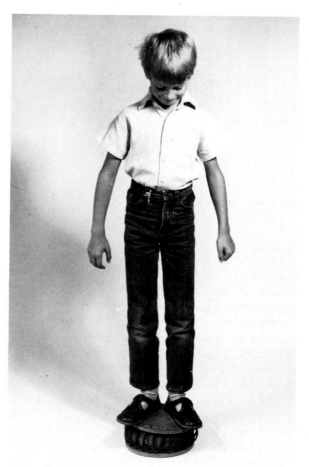

Fig. 23.4B The design can withstand considerable vertical loads.

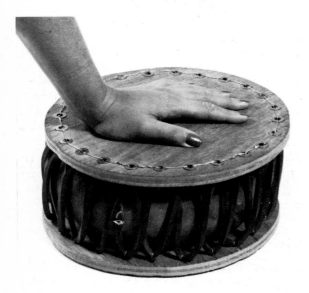

Fig. 23.4A A model of the intervertebral disc constructed from a football bladder laced with strands of rubber.

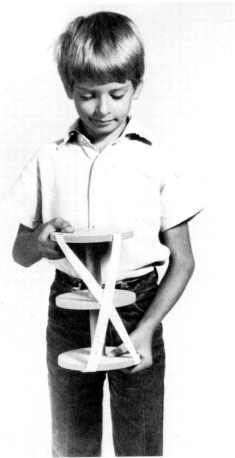

Fig. 23.5A   An elastic model of the alternating direction of the annular fibres.

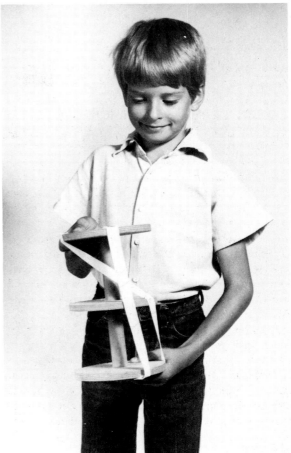

Fig. 23.5B   Rotation of the model will relax one layer at the expense of stretching the next layer, perhaps to failure.

to the function of the spine would not only reinforce the physics, but focus on the importance of the spine, (Fig. 23.6).

3. We do not truly learn until we apply what we have been taught. As practice produces the musician or sportsman, so only repetitive instruction can be expected to produce skilled handling and lifting techniques. Teachers of physical education are in a unique position to show, and train the young as week by week they reinforce what has been learnt in the classroom, demonstrating and correcting as the children lift and move apparatus about the gymnasium. They can instil a pride of achievement in their charges, that instead of being 'weak' if they cannot move a heavy weight, they are skilled when they learn how to lift. Perhaps the sport of weight lifting should be encouraged.

At local level, it is possible to arouse enthusiasm amongst teachers for this multi-disciplinary approach to back education. We conduct a seminar twice yearly for teachers of biology, physics and physical education, and in some schools this programme is being applied. There is no evidence yet that it will affect the incidence of back pain, but it is not unreasonable, and it may offer a way forward to reduce a major sickness problem in our society.

Educating the recruit

The heavy manual worker is 50 per cent more likely to experience back pain than the sedentary worker, 100 per cent more likely to visit his general practitioner with back pain, and 200 per cent more likely to be off work with back pain. It would seem

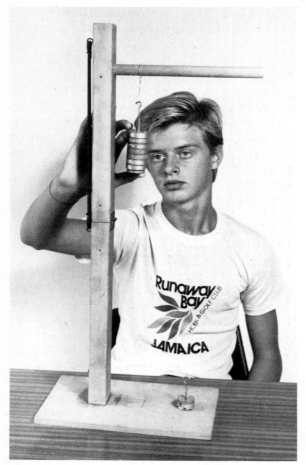

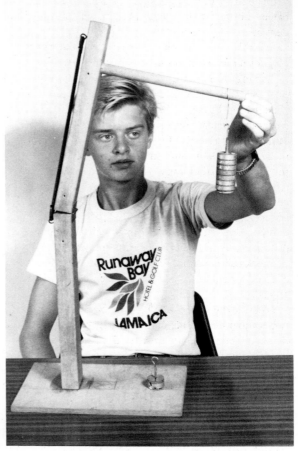

Fig. 23.6A A system of levers demonstrates that a structure can be stable if the load is close to the fulcrum.

Fig. 23.6B The same load at a distance from the fulcrum becomes unstable. (Models constructed by Dr. D. Ottewell.)

sensible to offer some teaching programme to recruits entering heavy manual industries, in the hope that they may take reasonable care with their backs. Many industries now give instruction in safe handling techniques, with talks, films and demonstrations, reinforced by in-service training. The value of such training programmes is still dubious, and opinions vary about its effects. Probably recruits who have no experience of back pain themselves, remember only for a short period information gathered at a 'Back School'. It is the established worker with a personal knowledge of back pain who will continue to apply the principles he has learnt.

Educating the back pain sufferer — The Back School: How can he avoid the next attack? How can

he keep at work without repeated periods of absenteeism? It may be done if he is fully informed about the types of stress that injure the spine, and is prepared to apply this in day to day activities. The hospital based 'Back School' is the best place for this education.

How to prevent the next attack is the most important advice we can offer. This present attack will generally settle in spite of us, but the next episode depends very much on whether we can generate new attitudes. For this reason clincians are tending to offer a 'Back School' programmme, rather than using resources and time on dubious therapeutic methods (Bergquist-Ullman and Larsson, 1977 and Williams, 1977, Attix and Tate, 1979, Fisk et al, 1983). The doctor can discuss the problem, present management and prognosis but cannot spend two or three hours with each patient explaining and demonstrating the correct use of the spine. This is the role of the 'Back School', presented by physiotherapists or occupational therapists.

Starting in Scandinavia, the 'Back School' concept has spread across the industrialised world (Zachrisson-Forsell 1972). There is no rigid structure, each department offering instruction tailored to the needs of the local community (Pawlicki et al, 1982). In our situation men are generally prepared to visit on only two occasions, whilst women will attend on three or four. The size of the class is generally six, and it helps if the participants in the group have similar intellectual ability.

What does the 'Back School' seek to achieve? To provide the patient with information about back pain of mechanical origin, how to manage recurrent and chronic pain, and how to reduce the incidence of attacks.

What is the content? We start by passing round a few lumbar vertebrae, and describe the vertebrae and discs, muscles and ligaments, the lumbar roots and cauda equina. The function of the spine is explained and how it can be abused (Fig. 23.5). Disc protrusions and degenerative change is described, and the vulnerability of the nerve roots in later life. The probable cause of the patient's pain is known to the physiotherapist, and she asks the patient if the pain mechanism described by the doctor has been understood. They are shown how to relax, when in sufficient pain, either on their side or with the knees and hips flexed on a stool, and told how to cope with an acute attack of back pain.

Correct lifting techniques are demonstrated and practised at the first session and reassessed, corrected and practised again at each subsequent session. Advice is offered about posture and the every day activities of lying, sitting, standing, reaching, crouching, twisting, pushing and pulling and how these can be accomplished with the minimum of spinal stress. Each patient is encouraged to contribute with questions and observations. They are taken individually through a normal day, and ways are sought to modify activities to reduce the stress on the spine. Anything that might be relevant to the spine is on the agenda. The physiotherapist tries to share the known facts but readily admits the large areas of continuing ignorance.

Some Back Schools will incorporate exercises into the programme (White 1983). A strong back is not possible with inadequate muscles, but we have yet to identify which patient will benefit from specific exercises.

One may argue theoretically that one posture is less stressful to the spine than another but there is little scientific proof that specific postures relieve backache. It makes sense that pain producing postures should be avoided but these may be very specific for individual patients. One cannot escape the view that certain individuals hold a 'good posture', but we have difficulty in defining what is good, and explaining why it is beter than another. Advocates of the Alexander technique attempt to inhibit poor postural habits (Gelb 1981); this may not affect back pain, but it looks good.

What are the results? It is difficult to present any claims that 'Back Schools' are dramatically effective. It is difficult to measure meaningful parameters and for comparable groups. Our own attempts comparing patients who attended the 'Back School' with defaulters, showed in fact that the non-attenders were just as satisfied. They returned to work as quickly, and had as little trouble over the subsequent year as the attenders. 'Back School' education however does seem to make good sense, it seems to meet the needs of many patients seeking medical help, and it does drop the anxiety level of many bewildered patients who have suffered with back pain for a long time with no-one attempting to explain the problem to them.

Rehabilitation

The natural history of most episodes of back pain encourages physicians to be more active in advocating a patient's return to work. Patients should be convinced that strict bed rest is usually necessary for only a few days after an acute episode, and then gradual increase in activity helps a functional recovery. A few patients benefit from residential rehabilitation in their progress to return to work, with the psychological and physical stimulus of competitive group therapy. They should be helped to return to work gradually and gently, preferably to an environment that is kind to the back. Such concepts need the support of social workers, employers and politicians (Nachemson, 1983). Alternatively, a long period of enforced rest, with no hope of work ultimately, is counter productive to re-developing a healthy back.

Education of the chronic sufferer

Self-help groups have developed over recent years to support patients and their families with many different medical problems (Gunn, 1984). Self-help groups are usually originated by people with some common problem where existing services and facilities are seen as unsatisfactory (Williamson and Danaker, 1978), and this is certainly true for some chronic back pain sufferers. There are many such groups now in the United Kingdom (Mansted 1980). They have common objectives:

1. To provide a venue for back-pain sufferers and their families to meet together and mutually improve their understanding of back pain and its management. The meetings are regular, friendly and informal, with a strong medical support, but a lay organisation. Those who appreciate such a group are often the middle aged who at least have found others who understand their predicament. Many distressed patients find support from such a group, where traditional management has failed. Perhaps they have met for the first time someone else like themselves. Talking out the problem and sharing experiences does not necessarily reduce the pain, but it can reduce the anxiety. One in ten back pain sufferers offered a self-help group may actually attend (Webb, 1982) but two-thirds of the group do admit to benefit.

2. To promote an understanding of back pain prevention in the local community. The drive of a well organised lay group can alert the community to its responsibility in back care, in industry, education and the wider society. Health education and preventive policies cannot be imposed on a community but they become effective by a one to one contact (Williams, 1984). Who better to make that contact at local level, but the informed patient, backed by doctors, physiotherapists and health workers.

3. To raise funds for local and national research. The appeal of back pain is less emotive than cancer, the illnesses of children, the elderly and the crippled. Self-help groups recognise the dearth of back pain research.

3. Identification of the individual at risk

Some individuals working in the same environment, subjecting their backs to identical stresses, are at greater risk than others of sustaining a back injury. Twenty per cent of coal miners can work underground lifting excessive loads in unacceptable positions, and never experience back pain, yet a colleague may leave the industry after only a few years and become a 'back cripple' for life. What is the difference? There are probably many factors:

a. The shape and size of the vertebral canal. Our own studies using ultrasound suggest that individuals with small sagittal diameters of the central lumbar vertebral canal are prone to develop low back pain. They are more likely to attend hospital (Porter et al, 1980) to be admitted and to have spinal surgery than subjects with deeper canals. The small canal with a trefoil shape is a particularly sinister combination if that canal is compromised by a disc protrusion, by osteophytic degenerative change or by segmental instability. It is necessary to have a relatively inexpensive and non-invasive method of identifying the canal's size and shape and ultrasound does appear to have the potential needed for screening. By contrast, radiographs have no pre-employment prediction value (La Rocca and Macnab, 1969).

b. Pre-employment strength testing. Chaffin has found a correlation between the ability of a man's back to stand up to the demands of his work, and his strength for the task (Chaffin and Park, 1973, and Chaffin et al, 1978). He has designed apparatus to record dynamic strength testing, and this may have an application in pre-employment screening (Troup, 1979, Beiring Sorensen, 1984). However, men with a pre-existing history of back pain will have reduced muscle strength, will be prone to further back pain, and unless excluded from any prospective series, they will invalidate the results.

c. The best predictor of back pain is a previous history (Roland et al, 1983, Lloyd and Troup, 1983 and Drinkall et al, 1984). A man is a poor risk entering a heavy labouring industry with a previous history of back pain, but this is an insensitive measure for young recruits.

d. The presence of abnormal signs Lloyd and Troup (1983) recorded that subjects with reduced straight leg raising were more likely to have subsequent absenteeism due to back pain. This reflects a pre-existing spinal pathology, and although a useful observation when recruiting older subjects, it is not particularly helpful when recruiting the young.

e. Anthropometry. Lawrence (1955) suggested that taller miners were prone to develop back pain, and Kelsey (1975) noted that taller women who had had multiple full term pregnancies were at risk. Merriam et al (1983) in a careful anthropometric study concluded that the pelvic height was significantly related to the incidence of back pain. Perhaps this with other body measurements may become a useful predictor but it requires further study when other epidemiological data suggests that neither height nor weight are associated risk factors for back pain (Buckle, 1983).

f. The family history. There is circumstantial evidence that the family history is important. There are many families where each member suffers from disabling back pain, often requiring similar surgical procedures. It would not be unreasonable to expect inheritance to affect the morphology of the vertebral canal, the resilience of the disc and the tendency to develop degenerative change, but apart from ankylosing spondylitis, there is no proven genetic association with back pain.

Our own studies suggest a familial relationship in 50 patients who had disc excision, 48 of their first degree relatives having significant low back pain. There were only 18 first degree relatives with back pain of 50 matched control subjects.

g. Tendency to develop abnormal pain behaviour. It is possible to identify patients exhibiting abnormal pain behaviour and these attend their general practitioner with various conditions many times above the average attendance rate. They find their way to many hospital departments. The women visit gynaecologists for a hysterectomy, frequent the dieticians and complain of back pain. They have tomes of medical notes and bulging packets of radiographs. They describe inappropriate symptoms, exhibit inappropriate signs and are resistant to treatment. Their rate of absenteeism from work is high, from all conditions as well as back pain. They feel pain and who can contradict them.

It would be helpful if such individuals could be identified in early adult life, to protect themselves from injuries of heavy manual work, their employers from absenteeism and their doctors from offering them harmful investigations and treatment.

The imprinting of abnormal pain behaviour will be present in early life (Melzack, 1973, Letham et al, 1983) but can it be recognised? One may speculate that a good history, a record of school absenteeism and a suitable psychological questionnaire would help.

We are at present only at the earliest stages of identifying risk factors, but we may soon be able to combine several factors and suggest the probability of a young adult eventually suffering from back pain. The ethics of screening is complex (Richardson 1984) but we accept that a certain acuity of vision is necessary for a pilot, and that a coal face worker requires good hearing. A strong spine is a requisite for the manual worker in a stressful environment, to protect him, his family and his employer from the complex physical and social distress of back pain. Where the environment cannot be changed and where education has its limitations the back pain problem will be reduced if the man is matched to the job. The size of the back pain problem, and our limitations in effectively treating it, makes prevention a priority.

REFERENCES

Attix E A, Tate M A 1979 Low back school: a conservative method for the treatment of low back pain. Journal of the Mississippi State Medical Association: 20, 4

Bergquist-Ullman M, Larson U 1977 Acute low back pain in industry: a controlled prospective study with special reference to therapy and compounding factors. Act Orthopaedica Scandinavia suppl. 170

Berry H, Bloom B, Hamilton E B D, Swinson 1981 Naproxen sodium, diflunisal and placebo in the treatment of chronic back pain. Annals of the Rheumatic Diseases 41: 129–132

Biering-Sorensen F 1984 Physical measurements as risk indicators for low back trouble over a one year period. Spine 9: 106–119

Buckle P 1983 A multi-disciplinary investigation of factors associated with low back pain. Ph.D. thesis Cranfield Institute of Technology, Bedfordshire.

Chaffin D B, Park K S 1973 A longitudinal study of low back pain as associated with occupational weight lifting factors. American Industrial Hyg. Assoc. Journal 34: 513–525

Chaffin D B, Herrin G D, Keyserling W M 1978 Pre-employment strength testing: an updated position. Journal of Occupational Medicine 20: 403

Coxhead C E, Inskip H, Meade T W, North W R S, Troup J D G 1981 Multicentric trial of physiotherapy and the management of sciatic symptoms. The Lancet 1981, 1065–1068

Davis P R, Stubbs D A 1976 A method of establishing safe handling forces in working situations. Symposium on safety in manual materials handling at Suny, Buffalo, organised by National Institute of Occupational Safety and Health

Davis P R, Stubbs D 1977 Radio Pills: their use in monitoring back stress. Journal of Medical Engineering and Technology 1: 209–212

Deyo R A 1983 Conservative therapy for low back pain: distinguishing useful from useless therapy. JAMA 205: 1057–1062

Doran D M L, Newell D J 1975 Manipulation in treatment of low back pain: a multicentric study. British Medical Journal 2: 161–164

Drinkall J N, Porter R W, Hibbert C S, Evans C 1984 The value of ultrasonic measurement of the spinal canal diameter in general practice. British Medical Journal 288: 121–122

Edwards B C 1969 Low back pain and pain resulting from lumbar spine conditions. A comparison of treatment results. Australian Journal of Physiotherapy 15: 104–109

Fiddler M W, Plasmans C M T 1983 The effect of four types of support on the segmental mobility of the lumbosacral spine. Journal of Bone and Joint Surgery, 65–A: 943–947

Fisk, J R, DiMonte P, Courington S McK 1983 Back Schools: past, present and future. Clinical Orthopaedics and Related Research 179: 18–23

Gelb M 1981 Body Learning. An introduction to the Alexander Technique. Aurum Press Limited, 11 Garrick Street, London

Gunn A D G 1984 Self Help. British Medical Journal 288: 1024–1025

Kelsey J L 1975 An epidemiological study of acute herniated lumbar intervertebral discs. Rheumatology and Rehabilitation 14: 144–159

La Rocca H, Macnab I 1969 Value of pre-employment radiographic assessment of the lumbar spine. Journal of the Canadian Medical Association 101: 49–54

Lawrence J S 1955 Rheumatism in coal miners. British Journal of Industrial Medicine 12: 249–261

Leskinen T P J, Stalhammar H R, Kuorinka I A A 1983 A dynamic analysis of spinal compression with different lifting techniques. Ergonomics 26: 595–604

Letham J, Slade P D, Troup J D G, Bentley G 1983. Outline of a fear-avoidance model of exaggerated pain perception. Behaviour Research Therapy 21: 401–408

Lewith G T, Turner G M T 1982 Retrospective analysis of the management of acute low back pain. Practitioner 226: 1614–1618

Lloyd P, Allan M C, Haggerty A, Lee M E, Scrivenger M, Peake S 1979 Avoiding low back injury among nurses. Report of Royal College of Nursing of the United Kingdom

Lloyd D C E F, Troup J D C 1983 Recurrent back pain and its prediction. Journal of Society of Occupational Medicine 33: 66–74

Lumsden R M and Morris J M 1968 An in vivo study of axial rotation and immobilisation at the lumbo sacral joint. Journal of Bone and Joint Surgery 50–A: 1591–1602

McKenzie R A 1981 The Lumbar Spine. Mechanical diagnosis and therapy. Spinal Publications Limited, PO Box 2, Waikanae, New Zealand

Manning D P, Shannon H S 1979 Injuries of the lumbosacral region in a gear box factory. Journal of Society of Occupational Medicine 29: 144–148

Manstead S K 1979 Despair or self-help: the choice is yours. Back Pain Association, 33 Park Road, Teddington, Middlesex.

Melzack R 1973 The puzzle of pain. Penguin Books Ltd, Middlesex, England

Merriam W F, Burwell R G, Mulholland R C, Pearson J C G, Webb J K 1983 A study revealing a tall pelvis in subjects with low back pain. Journal of Bone and Joint Surgery. 65–B: 153–156

Million R, Nilsen K H, Jayson M I V, Baker R D 1981 Evaluation of low back pain and assessment of lumbar corsets with and without back supports. Annals of the Rheumatic Diseases 40: 449–454

Morrison M C T 1983 The best back to manipulate? Annals of the Royal College of Surgeons of England 66: 52–53

Nachemson A, Elfstrom G 1970 Intravital dynamic pressure measurements in lumbar discs: a study of common movements, manoeuvres and exercises. Almqvist and Wilksell, Stockholm

Nachemson A 1983 Work for all. Clinical Orthopaedics and Related Research 179: 77–85

Norton P L, Brown T 1957 The immobilizing efficiency of back braces. Their effect on the posture and motion of the lumbosacral spine. Journal of Bone and Joint Surgery 39–A: 111–138

Otun E O, Henrich I, Anderson J A D and Crooks J 1984 'Padas' an ambulatory electronic system to monitor and evaluate factors relating to back pain at work. Journal of Ergonomics 27: 268–271.

Pawlicki R E, Gil K M, Jopling C A, Bettinger R, Stevenson J M 1982 The low back school: a new palliative approach to low back pain. The West Virginia Medical Journal 78, 10, 249–251

Porter R W, Hibbert C, Wellman P, Langton C 1980 The shape and the size of the lumbar spinal canal. Proceedings of the Institute of Mechanical Engineers

Richardson I M 1984 Screening for Health. British Medical Journal 288: 1887–1888

Roland M O, Morrell D C, Morris R W 1983 Can general practitioners predict the outcome of episodes of back pain? British Medical Journal 286: 523–525

Scholey M 1983 Back stress: the effects of training nurses to lift patients in a clinical situation. Int. Journal Nurs. Stud 20: 1: 1–13

Schultz A B, Andersson G B J, Haderspeck K, Ortengren R, Nordin M, Bjork R 1982 Analysis and measurement of lumbar trunk loads in tasks involving bends and twists. Journal of Biomechanics 15: 669–675

Sims-Williams H, Jayson M I, Baddeley N 1978 Small spinal fractures in back pain patients. Annals of the Rheumatic Diseases 37: 262–265

Stubbs D A, Buckle P W, Hudson M P, Rivers P M, Worringham R J 1983 Back pain in the nursing profession, Part 1. Epidemiology and pilot methodology. Ergonomics 26: 8: 755–765

Troup J D G 1977, Dynamic factors in the analysis of the stoop and crouch lifting matters. Orthopaedic Clinics of North America 8: 201–209

Troup J D G 1979 Biomechanics of the vertebral column. Physiotherapy 65: 238–244

Troup J D G 1981 Back pain in industry: a prospective survey. Spine 6: 61–69

Webb P 1982 Back to self care? Physiotherapy 68: 295–297

Weber H 1973 Traction therapy in sciatica due to disc prolapse. Journal of Oslo City Hospital 23: 167–176

Weber H 1980 Comparison of the effect of diazepam and levomepromazine on pain in patients with acute lumbago-sciatica. Journal of the Oslo City Hospitals 30: 65–68

Weber H, Aasand G 1980 The effect of phenylbutazone on patients with acute lumbago-sciatica. A double blind trial. Journal of the Oslo City Hospitals 30: 69–72

White A H 1983 Back school and other conservative approaches to low back pain. The C V Mosby Company St. Louis, Toronto, London.

Williams B T 1984 Are public health education campaigns worthwhile? British Medical Journal 288: 170–171

Williams S J 1977 Back School. Physiotherapy 63: 90

Williamson and Danaker 1978 Self care in health, Groom Helm, London

Zachrisson-Forsell M 1972 Low back pain school. Danderyds Hospital, Sweden

Index